funny
little
pregnant
things

funny little pregnant things

(the good, the bad and
the just plain gross
things about pregnancy that other
books aren't going to tell you)

emily doherty

SparkPress

Published by SparkPress, a BookSparks imprint,
A division of SparkPoint Studio, LLC
Tempe, Arizona, USA, 85281
www.sparkpointstudio.com

ISBN: 978-1-940716-58-9 (pbk)
ISBN: 978-1-940716-57-2 (ebk)
LCCN: 2015953520

Cover design © Julie Metz, Ltd./metzdesign.com
Cover photo © Neil Beckerman/Getty Images
Author photo © Rammelkamp Foto
Interior design by Tabitha Lahr

Please note that suggestions in this book are not meant to replace the
proper role of a nutritionist, doctor, midwife, or other health care provider.
If you think you have a serious problem with your pregnancy, please seek
professional help. This book is not intended as a substitute for the medical
advice of physicians. The reader should regularly consult a physician in
matters relating to his/her health and particularly with respect to any
symptoms that may require diagnosis or medical attention.

To my husband, Patrick: without you this book could never have been written. You do an amazing job raising our children. I am in awe of you every day. Thanks for keeping the laughter in our house alive.

contents

(Introduction)

Hi there! I want to start by letting you know that I am not a doctor—or any sort of professional when it comes to babies—and will not be giving any medical advice in this book. So if you've picked it up because you want technical explanations for why you are sweating through your clothes and every sheet you own . . . you may want to get a different book.

Also keep in mind this book is not designed to tell you the "best" way to do anything. Before, during, and after your pregnancy, you'll have plenty of people telling you, "This is how I did it, and my way is, in fact, the best way." But the truth is, all pregnancies are different, and so are the babies they produce; it follows, then, that one method of preparation may work for one baby and not the next. And besides, they—whoever "they" are—change the rules all the time anyway. "Microwave your deli meat . . . Never mind, just use caution while eating." *Good, 'cause I wasn't going to do that anyway.* "Gain as much weight as you want while you're pregnant . . . actually, we're only going to budget you twenty pounds." *Whoops, too late!* "Have a martini and a cigarette, it will help you relax . . . er, actually, we got that one wrong, steer clear of the booze and smoke!" *Yeah, no sh*t Sherlock.*

So what exactly *is* this book—and why, as a working mom with a two-year-old and a three-week-old, have I decided to write it?

First, the why. Here's the thing: As a mom-to-be, I read a few of the prerequisite pregnancy books, and although I picked up some facts from them, I couldn't get over how *dull* they were. When Chapter 3 of the fourth book I attempted to slog through let me know that my baby was now the size of a lemon, I gave up. *Is there actual practicality in knowing that my child resembles a certain type of fruit?* I wondered. *Where's the good stuff?*

Besides how boring those books were, they were also incomplete. Now that I've had two babies, I understand just how many little details they left out—details that you only know if you've delivered a child; details that are very, very important. (Not one of those books, for example, told me that I should be prepared to get breast milk all over everything I owned after I gave birth!)

At least provide me with a pregnancy book with some humour, I thought. *Then maybe I can make it to Chapter 6 and not be super annoyed when you tell me that my baby now resembles a melon.*

So this book is for women like me—moms-to-be who want some realistic tips about what to expect from pregnancy without being bored to tears along the way. Here you will find accounts of the ridiculous things you'll likely encounter while pregnant, including the good, the bad, and the often gross stuff that people so conveniently forget to mention to you when you first decide to have a child.

In that spirit, let me get one of the big ones out in the open right now: There is a greater-than-average chance that you will sh*t yourself while giving birth. And there's nothing you can do about it. If it's gonna happen, it's gonna happen.

Pregnancy . . . anyone who said it would be easy (or pretty) was a big, fat liar.

PART ONE:

(The Beginning)

If you bought this book you are probably already preggo—but in the event that you aren't, let's just start with the initial step of actually getting pregnant, and go all the way to D-Day (also known as "delivery day").

I distinctly remember my first sexual education class in middle school. It was incredibly awkward because they split up the boys and the girls and they required your parents to sign a permission slip in advance for you to even attend.

During the class we were taught mostly about bodily changes like "breast buds" (whoever named that term should be fired), body odor, and leg hair; but we also got our first introduction to how babies are "made." They led us to believe that pretty much all a boy had to do was breathe on you and you would become pregnant. My best friend at the time was a boy, so this scared the living daylights out of me.

Later on, in high school, I had to attend another round of sexual education classes, and although these were much more progressive in their messaging, the overall thesis on how easy it was to have a baby didn't change. Unless you wore a condom or were taking birth control, they told us, unprotected sex at any time was pretty much guaranteed to lead to the production of a baby.

You may be shocked, like I was, to know that this is a gross overstatement. Your body can't just get pregnant any time a bunch of semen takes a tour of your vagina. You can only really conceive a child during the week leading up to ovulation. This tends to be a five- to seven-day window for most women. If you have sex outside of that time frame, your body has missed its chance, and will have to wait till the next cycle to try again. Great odds if you just had sex in the backseat of a car and the condom broke, but tough if you are actually trying to make a baby.

I mention all of this not to give the green light to a bunch of lusty teenagers (p.s., unlike pregnancy, STDs can happen at any time), but to give a heads up to the couples who are "trying" for a child. Getting pregnant is not as easy as you may think, and it can take a long time for many people.

If you're having trouble getting pregnant, try to take the stress out of the process. There are way too many calendaring systems and timing techniques out there. Dropping everything to have sex every time your phone app notifies you it's "go time" is enough to drive anyone crazy. Try to relax a bit and let nature take its course.

If you've been trying for a while and are still having trouble with conception, you may need to consult a doctor. Infertility is very common in both men and women; you are not alone.

And so we begin.

(Taking the Test)

Taking a pregnancy test, for most people, means going to your local pharmacy and coughing up the ten bucks it costs to buy one off the shelf. Warning: You are about to be royally ripped off. The pregnancy test is the first (though by no means the last) scam of the birthing industry. There is no way that those glorified pieces of plastic should cost anywhere near ten dollars, but they do. And you rarely just buy one of them.

Our first child was a surprise, so by the time I took a pregnancy test I was doing it to confirm something I had pretty much figured out already. So in this case I actually did only buy one. (Guess that's the upside to an unplanned pregnancy!) When it came to our second child, however, we were actively trying, which meant that every time I felt even the glimmer of a hot flash or nausea, I would go running to the pharmacy to purchase a new test.

The time I was absolutely sure I was pregnant was during the summer of 2013, when we were "trying" for a second baby. All of the signs were there: I was sweating nonstop, my stomach was doing flip-flops, and I was in constant bitch mode. Aiding my conception confidence was the fact that I had recently decided I was going to increase my chances of becoming pregnant by making sex an Olympic event—the Sex Capades. All month long I had "encouraged" (the words "made" or "pressured" are probably more accurate, but they also sound very inappropriate) my husband to have sex with me.

Here are some of the events we competed in:

- **The Morning Romp and Roll:** I would wait for him to wake up, then roll on top of him, hissing, "Quick let's do this before the baby (our first born) wakes up!"

- **The Shower In and Out:** I would wait for him to turn on the shower, then sneak in there after him—"Quick, before the water gets cold!"

- **The Lunch and Lust:** When he came into the kitchen to eat, I'd pounce—"Oh you have time for a sandwich? Then you have time for baby making too. Quick, before I have to go back to work!"

- **The Fold and Fu*k:** I would lure him into the laundry room—"Quick, let's have sex and then you can help me fold the laundry!" (This one had double advantages.)

One time we were driving somewhere, and I became so adamant that sex had to happen immediately that we pulled into a secluded area and hopped into the backseat of our car ("Quick, before we get arrested!"). Fun, but I swear those backseats have shrunk since high school.

(Side note for my male readers: I know that sex multiple times a day sounds like a very fun idea. Unfortunately, your fantasies of a real-life Skinemax experience will fade away when you realize that your pregnancy-crazed wife is really just using you so she can hijack your semen. I recommend not taking this too personally—and also purchasing a Costco-sized jar of lubricant.)

After a month of competing in the Sex Capades, my surefire pregnancy symptoms started showing up, and I was ready to receive my medal. I perched over the toilet and peed on the stick, and as I waited for the golden results, I swore I could hear the national anthem being played in the background. *And the medal goes to . . . not pregnant?? What the hell!*

There went another ten bucks down the toilet. Plus, I thought I might have pulled my groin from all the sex. But still I persevered.

The tricky part about early pregnancy symptoms is that they are very similar to those you likely encounter prior to getting your period each month. So when you get it wrong, not only do you end up feeling bummed that you are not pregnant, you also have to then spend the next few days bleeding like a stuck pig, waiting impatiently to be able to start the baby-making process all over again.

Even though I gave us a participation medal for effort, that time, like so many others, was a false alarm. I eventually stopped being so hell-bent on getting pregnant and decided to let nature take its course, which did the trick.

I'm glad my husband never caught on to how many of those pregnancy tests I actually bought while trying to have a second baby, because I was basically peeing money away for weeks. Luckily, eighty dollars and two blue lines later we were finally pregnant again, and the constant dashes to the pharmacy ended.

(Side note: Just like the wedding industry, the baby industry will take every opportunity to overcharge eager newbies. And it's because expecting mothers—and their family members, and their friends—tend to go baby crazy the second the words "I'm pregnant" are voiced. The industry knows this, and will gladly help everyone involved fulfill your dreams of buying everything you "need" at a fantastically high price. Start saving now; the pee stick is just the beginning.)

Okay, back to the process. You get home, you go into the bathroom, and you open your test. First thing's first: Read the directions! Pregnancy tests are like scratch tickets—you have to read carefully to see what it takes to win. Sometimes you are winner if you see one line, sometimes it's two, and if you're really lucky your pee may even make a smiley face appear! Make sure you understand what a positive/negative is going to look like before you get started; it's no fun getting them confused.

When you're ready, pull down your pants and assume the awkward hover-over-the-toilet-squatting-position. The next step after this is tricky: you have to reach your hand between your legs and try to pee on an inch-long absorbent strip that you can't see.

It would be nice if our pee came out slowly, in a steady, straight stream; however, as all non-penis bearers know, this is seldom the case. So no, your pregnancy test will not be a neat and tidy experience. It will be a messy one. It is very likely that your pee will spray out to the sides—hitting the strip, yes, but also hitting the hand you're using to hold the test. Don't worry: peeing on yourself while taking a pregnancy test is perfectly normal, and it's nothing to fret about—or to be embarrassed about. Just wash your hands when you're done and pretend it never happened.

If you are completely appalled by this idea and want

to avoid "urine hand," here are a few things you can try to stay dry:

1. **The head-between-your-legs method:** Instead of doing the blind spray, try leaning forward and looking down between your legs as you pee. This will allow you to see where and what you are peeing on. Be careful, though, because this may make you dizzy; the last thing you need is to fall forward and hit your head while executing this move. I'd rather get urine hand than a concussion, personally.

2. **Peeing into a cup:** A cup's wide diameter makes it easier to contain the shower-like stream women produce. Once you've filled your cup, dip your test in for the same amount of time you were supposed to spend peeing on it.

3. **Wearing gloves:** This one is self-explanatory. (Right?)

I ended up doing a combo. I would start with my head between my legs to line up the stick properly. Then, before I got too dizzy, I would look straight ahead and blindly pee. This method assured me that I would hit the stick, but left to chance whether my pee would hit my hand as well. I am always in the mood for a little pregnancy test roulette.

After you've peed on the stick (whichever method you've used to do it), the waiting game begins. At this point, you are probably thinking one of two things: "Please, God, let me be pregnant" or "No whammies, no whammies, no whammies!"

Whatever result you're hoping for, if that test reads positive, life as you know it is about to change forever. Some of those changes are absolutely amazing—like the fact that you are now growing an actual human being inside of you; and some of those changes are incredibly scary—like knowing that baby inside you is getting a lot bigger, and at some point, he or she is going to have to come out of what is, comparatively, a very tiny hole.

(Don't Tell the World
Just Yet)

Once you find out you're pregnant, you'll have the urge to tell everyone and their mother about it—and with today's technology, that is actually possible. While I totally sympathize with that urge, I have some disappointing news for you: you should resist it.

When my doctor told me there was about a one-in-five chance of having a miscarriage as a healthy young adult, and that the odds just get worse as you age, I was shocked. I had no clue how common miscarriages were, especially with your first child. Learning this, I finally understood why so many women keep quiet about their pregnancies until way after they find out they have a bun in the oven.

In my case, my mother was the only person we told about the positive pregnancy test. After hearing the miscarriage statistics, had we told more, I would have bolted from the OB's office to shut down all of my social media accounts until the coast was clear.

The rule of thumb is to wait until you have made it past your first twelve weeks. If everything is still normal by then, go ahead and update your status; I'm sure you'll have at least seventy-three likes within minutes! But until your doctor tells you you're in the clear, I wouldn't recommend telling anyone (besides your partner, of course, and maybe your best friend). Better safe than sorry!

(Naming Your Child)

If you don't have a family name you want to pass on to the next generation, choosing your baby's name can be very difficult. Out of the thousands of possibilities, you have to narrow it down to one name—a single title that will identify your child for the rest of his or her life.

No pressure, right?

When we found out we were pregnant, my husband and I went out and bought a baby name book, hoping for a little guidance. In hindsight, this was not our best move—*"Oh you don't know what to name your child? Here are 56,000 names to choose from!"* You wouldn't believe the variety you find in those books: Ham, Bojo, Quintessence,

Mimosa, Siobhan, Aoife, *Speedracer*—out of control! We couldn't even pronounce half of the names listed. Total baby-naming overload. (PS. Siobhan is actually a very pretty girl's name—definitely not phonetic, however.)

It took us my entire pregnancy to pick a name for our first son. By the final weeks before my due date, we had narrowed it down to two choices: one I liked, and one my husband liked more. We went back and forth on whose name was the better choice, and neither of us would budge. When I went into labor, we were still divided on the issue.

In almost all scenarios in life, the woman gets her way—especially when she's pregnant. But in this particular instance, the decision was made while I was lying on the operating table, post C-section, doped up to the extreme. I groggily peered up at my husband, and he just looked so amazing holding our firstborn. Voice full of awe, I said, "You name him." And he did.

I am 100 percent positive if I hadn't been loaded full of pain meds and caught up in the euphoria of just having delivered a baby, I would not have given in. But I couldn't exactly take it back once the drugs and adrenaline wore off.

When it comes to naming your baby, the best advice I can give you is the same advice I just gave you in the last chapter about what to do when you first find out you're pregnant: *keep it to yourself*. Once you come up with a name, however long it takes, do not tell anyone what it is until your baby is born. Why? Because revealing your baby's name before birth opens up the floor for comment—and people have all kinds of opinions when it comes to names, most of them negative:

> *"Oh, you're going with John? I like that name, it's nice and ordinary."*

> *"Sally? I love that name—it's the name of my parent's dog!"*

> *"Jeremy? I had a friend named Jeremy. We went to school together. I think he ended up in jail."*

> *"Colin? You're going to name your child after a butthole?"*

Need I say more?

Some people may have the good manners to *tell* you they like the name you've chosen, but half the time even these polite folks won't be able to hide their real feelings about it—if they're lying, their facial expression will give it away. And every time you have these conversations, you will feel bad, and maybe even rethink your decision.

When my friend Sarah was pregnant, she (smartly) refused to tell anyone but her sister what name she had picked out for the baby. She was literally on the delivery table, having contractions and in the midst of pushing, when her doctor asked what they were naming their daughter.

At this point, Sarah felt it was pretty safe to finally reveal the name—not a whole lot of time to change her mind anyway!—so she told him: "Ezrah."

The doctor stopped what he was doing, looked up from between her legs with a creased brow, and said, "Don't you know that's a Jewish boy's name?"

If I were Sarah, I would have removed my foot from the birthing stirrup and kicked him square in the face. I still don't understand how she held herself back.

Just wait—I swear, you won't regret it. Before your baby is born, people seem to think they have a vote when it comes to what you will name your child; but after your baby is born, they will only say favorable things about the name you've chosen (to your face, anyway).

PART TWO:

(The Holy Trinity)

Yay, you're pregnant! As you settle into this new phase of life, try not to think about the things you did to your body leading up to your pregnancy—like the shots you took at the bar the night you conceived. I actually found out I was pregnant with my first child the day after Halloween; you can imagine how horrified I felt knowing that, just hours before, I had been running the beer pong table dressed as a Ninja Turtle. But what I had to accept—what we all have to accept—is that it's too late to fret now. Odds are your baby is totally fine. (It's probably a good idea to put away the shot glasses and cigarettes going forward, though!)

Fortunately for my fellow Ninja Turtles—but unfortunately for me—none of them were also with child at the time. I became the first in our group of friends to become pregnant, which of course made me the guinea pig. I didn't know a whole lot about what to expect going into pregnancy. I was aware that certain things tended to happen at certain times, but I was completely in the dark about most of the day-to-day details. Turns out, the changes in your hormones—those teensy-weensy chemical messengers in your body that don't seem like they should be such a big deal—can do a real number on you. In fact, hormones are pretty much to blame for almost everything crazy that happens to you while you're pregnant, both emotionally and physically.

I don't want you to go into your first pregnancy as blindly as I went into mine. So, in the next part of this book, I have highlighted some of the more interesting, grotesque, and downright hysterical pregnancy-related changes that stood out to me during the forty weeks leading up to my firstborn's delivery. I have categorized this period of time and the symptoms that occur during it into three main stages. I like to refer to these stages as the "Holy Trinity": *Holy sh*t, I feel awful*; *Holy crap, I feel great*; and *Holy cow, get this baby out of me*. As you read through the next few chapters, you will understand exactly what I mean.

Let's dive in!

(Wet Dreams)

I am not referring to a nocturnal emission here; this, sadly, has nothing at all to do with sex. Not even close. No, what I'm referring to with this chapter title is one of the first things that tipped me off to go and take a pregnancy test: the amount of sweat I was producing at night.

I remember being away on business and waking up in my hotel room totally drenched. My clothes, the blankets, and the sheets were soaked through. It was as though I had been running a marathon in my sleep. But since I am not accustomed to doing any type of exercise while sleeping, and I had no idea that this was a potential pregnancy side effect, I jumped to a much more embarrassing conclusion—that I had channeled my inner toddler (or blacked out college freshman) and pissed the bed!

Luckily it didn't end up being pee (spoiler: stay tuned for later chapters when I actually *do* pee myself). It was just a very severe case of the night sweats.

Although disgusting, night sweats during pregnancy are 100 percent normal. All this moisture happens because of the flood of hormones raging through your body, particularly at the start of pregnancy, and there's not a whole lot you can do to stop it. There are, however, a few things that may help you out:

1. Start wearing loose-fitting clothing to bed—or, if you are up for it, just go ahead and sleep in the buff.

2. Sleep on top of a towel. This should keep the sweat on the towel and limit the amount of sheet laundering you will have to do.

3. If you and your partner share a double bed or smaller, one of you may want to spend some time on the couch until your body normalizes. (If that's not an option, at the very least be kind enough to purchase your partner a poncho so he or she can wake up dry!)

Since my husband refused to sleep anywhere but our bed, I went with the towels. I ended up lining my side of the bed each night. Then when I woke up in the middle of the night to go to the bathroom (again, refer to later chapters—this happened a lot!), I would swap the soaked towels out for dry ones. Our detergent bill went sky high—sorry, environment—but we made it through.

(It's 5:30 P.M., I Think I'll Go to Bed)

I was shocked at how tired I felt in the first three months of my pregnancy. In hindsight, though, it makes sense—my body was, after all, literally creating another human being. So when you can't even make it through dinner without falling asleep in the mashed potatoes, don't fight it; just go to bed. There will come a time (and it will come quite soon) when sleep will not be an option, so take advantage of the opportunity to get a little extra shut-eye while you can.

When the pregnancy exhaustion begins to set in, you

may want to give your partner a heads up that you are going to be kind of boring for the next few months.

With our firstborn, right up until the four-month mark, I was sleeping by 8:00 P.M. every night. And eight was actually quite the accomplishment. If I'd had it my way I would have been sleeping by six, but my husband was bored out of his mind, so he did everything he could to keep me going at least through dinnertime.

On the bright side, your dormancy can actually help your relationship. First of all, getting plenty of sleep can help reduce moodiness (I was a huge B.I.T.C.H. during both of my pregnancies. I blame my hormones and not my actual personality, but excuses aside, if I were my husband, I would have been begging me to just go to bed.) Rest up enough, and hopefully the bickering over whose turn it is to do the dishes will be kept to a minimum.

If your partner is a TV watcher with tastes different from your own, you crashing before prime time also means that they get to highjack the remote and watch whatever they want without you vetoing their choices. When I finally returned to a more adult bedtime routine, right around month number four, I checked the DVR and all of my shows had been replaced with golf, SportsCenter, and Seinfeld.

I didn't begrudge my husband his few months of TV dominance—not too much, anyway, especially since it didn't take long to get the DVR back to its former glory.

Within a day or two of vigilant reprogramming, balance was restored, and all was right with the world. Hello Gordon Ramsey, goodbye Kramer.

Final word here: Going to bed when your body is tired means everyone wins, so grab the PJs and hit the sack.

(It's 5:30 P.M., Why Can't I Go to Bed??)

If this is not your first child, you know that going to bed at five thirty is not a realistic plan no matter how tired you are. Unless your partner is a saint, you are most likely not going to find slumber until the rest of your family does.

My husband is a stay-at-home dad and pretty much amazing, but certainly not a saint. After watching our Energizer Bunny toddler all day, there were very few times while I was pregnant that he suggested I go lie down when I came home from work. As a result, getting to bed before 8:00 P.M.

was definitely not going to happen for me during pregnancy number two—which meant that during said pregnancy, I slowly began to turn into a sleep-deprived zombie.

After a few months of this, I knew I had to find an alternative. If I wasn't going to be allowed to nap at night, then I would have to seek out another time. It was either that or continue with the zombie thing and probably end up eating my family.

I first tried waking up in the morning with our son and going right back to sleep. I would set him up in the activity seat, turn on cartoons, and pass out on the couch. Genius, right? But this "wake and nap" method didn't last long. First of all, it's probably bad parenting. Second, if you have a toddler, you know that the assumption that your child is just going to sit there watching television while you sleep is just plain silly. All mine had to do was turn his head once and see me there on the couch—within sight but out of reach—and he would start yelling. Even the old blanket-over-the-head trick couldn't fool him. He knew I was there.

My final attempt to get some extra sleep was to find time to nap during the day. This sounds good on paper, but getting yourself to sleep in the middle of the day if you are not a "napper"—or if you work full-time—is no easy task. Luckily, I stumbled across a pretty neat solution one day when, sleep deprived and borderline desperate, I went on YouTube and looked up "sleep hypnosis power nap"—

and voilà! I found video after video featuring gentle voices meant to talk your body into relaxing and, eventually, into sleep. This method began to work so well for me that I had to start setting an alarm before I settled in to listen, just in case my body decided my "power" nap should be more like a three-hour slumber.

What to do if you work full-time, you ask? Well, I *was* working full-time—I just went ahead and took my naps anyway. When my afternoon slump hit, I headed out to my car, cracked the windows, leaned back the seat, and started one of the videos. I ended up spending thirty minutes to an hour each day sound asleep in a parking lot. Not my first choice of napping venue, but it was the only thing that made lasting till 8:00 P.M. at night doable.

Warning: If you are going to use your car as your personal crash pad, find a cool and safe location, and be sure to lock your doors. Also, try to make it clear that you're sleeping and not dead; I once fell into such a deep sleep during one of my naps that a concerned passerby knocked on my window to check on me and nearly scared the baby out of me!

("Morning" Sickness)

Ah, morning sickness. This symptom obviously falls under the "holy sh*t, I feel awful" time, but I find it to be a very misleading pregnancy term. Why do we only give the morning credit? With my second child, I was pretty much sick all day long. I felt like I had the flu—or, to be more accurate, I felt like the life was literally being sucked out of me. And it just went on . . . and on . . . and on.

The problem with morning sickness is that it usually occurs during the first trimester—a time when, if you have a job, you probably still have to go to work no matter how crummy you feel, and a time when you're also not ready to tell the world you are pregnant. If the latter is true for you, not only do you feel like crap, you also have to be good at making up stories on the fly to explain why you just threw up on your coworker's shoes. Some white lies that may work: food poisoning, stomach bug, the flu, vertigo, someone snuck some ipecac into my morning coffee, too much tequila, etc. Warning: use the last one sparingly, or people will think you have an actual problem—which is probably worse than them just finding out that you're pregnant.

Another thing to do to prepare for feeling like crap is keep a sickness survival kit with you. Since I drive a lot for work, I started keeping the following items in my car: a trash can (to hold the occasional vomit), toothpaste and a toothbrush (to wash out the vomit), bottles of water (to wash out the toothpaste that washed out the vomit), and snacks (to replace what came out with the vomit).

Speaking of snacks, many women can reduce or eliminate the queasy feeling by eating a little something throughout the day. I found that saltines work wonders, but I recommend going for the low-salt variety—believe me, at this point you'll be retaining enough water as it is.

Here's a silver lining to keep in mind when you're racing to the bathroom for the fourth time in one day: Morning sickness can be a sign that your hormone levels are exactly where they should be. In fact, there is evidence that women who experience morning sickness are less likely to miscarry. So while you're heaving up that oatmeal, take comfort in the fact that your baby is probably feeling great.

With any luck, by month four the sickness should subside. In my case the sickness went away overnight. I remember waking up one morning, ready for the stomach churning to begin, and it just didn't. Just like that, I went from feeling awful to feeling as close to normal as a girl with a rapidly expanding body could.

If you are one of the unlucky ones and are sick your entire pregnancy, let me just offer you my condolences in advance. It's going to be a long forty weeks. But I promise—it will be worth it.

(Dr. Jekyll and Mrs. Hyde)

Dear Patrick,

I am incredibly sorry for the way I treated you from October 2010 to June 2011. I don't know why I felt you could not do anything right or why I felt the need to either yell or cry to get my emotions across on a daily basis. Thank you for bearing with my erratic behavior and for not divorcing me.

Love,
The mother of your children, Emily

If you want your significant other to read any part of this book, this is probably the chapter you should point them to. Because some pregnancies may cause you to literally go *insane*, and that's something your partner needs to understand early on.

As with most of pregnancy's fun little side effects, those pesky hormones are to blame for the crazies you're going to feel leading up to giving birth, and they can completely change who you are as a person. I generally consider myself to be somewhat easygoing—or, at the very least, not a mean person—but when I was pregnant with my first child, I turned into Mrs. Hyde, with no Dr. Jekyll in sight. I'm pretty sure not a day went by that I didn't yell or cry, and my husband, as he was the only one at home with me, was the one who received the brunt of those hostile emotions.

The majority of my rage was focused on two areas: an obsession with having a clean house, and my husband's late-night outings with his friends. In normal times, these two issues would not cause any conflict in our home. My husband's generally a pretty clean guy, and honestly I like it when he spends time with buddies—it gives me time to watch all of the ridiculous, brain-draining Bravo shows he refuses to watch with me. But in pregnant times, dishes in the sink and a husband not home till 11:00 P.M. led to immediate rage. Do not pass go, do not collect one hundred dollars, go straight to yelling and crying pregnant wife mode.

The worst part (for him, anyway)? I didn't even realize until after I gave birth and my hormones chilled out a bit that I was behaving totally out of character. Poor Patrick.

The only advice I have here is 1) when these moments happen, try to remember that it's the hormones talking, and 2) keep in mind that these negative feelings are temporary, and they should go away just as quickly as they wash over you. Also, getting your endorphins going will help you be less of a bitch, so try and get out for some exercise on a regular basis. Try yoga—or, if you don't have the energy for yoga, just try meditation.

If none of these activities work or your negative mood continues far past your pregnancy, consult your doctor—you could be experiencing postpartum depression. I had this following both of my pregnancies. It is a very real thing, and usually requires real medical attention.

Significant others: If you are reading this, I am sorry for you in advance. There is really nothing you can do to appease an emotional pregnant woman. The best thing to do is go with the flow and don't take what she says to heart. Somewhere in there is the woman you wanted to sleep with and will want to continue to sleep with after your baby is born. If there is a pattern to her behavior or a time of day when she is at her worst, wait for that time . . . and hide.

(Cravings)

People you meet while pregnant will always ask you the same questions: *When are you due? Boy or girl? Do you have a name? Do you have any strange cravings?* Be prepared to answer these a hundred times. Personally, I got sick of saying the same thing over and over, so I started making up answers after a while: *I'm not pregnant, just fat. I am having twins, and their names will be Salt and Peppa—yes, named after the girl group. I also can't stop craving envelope glue.*

In reality, I never craved anything at all while pregnant, which came as a disappointment, because I think it is pretty cool that your body's preference for food can change as a result of having a bun in the oven. It also would have been an awesome excuse to eat as much junk food as possible. ("Honey, I need you to run the store for some ice cream and potato chips—no, not for me, for the baby!")

The truth is, instead of craving certain foods, I experienced the opposite: an adamant distaste for edible items that I would normally enjoy.

The first thing to go was gum. I have a job that requires that I talk to people, up close and in person, all day, so I always used to travel with a pack—but as soon as I got pregnant, I became absolutely repulsed by all chewing gum. I don't know if it was the flavor or the texture that initially turned me off, but just like that I couldn't even smell it without gagging. To this day, I rarely chew gum.

The second thing to go was coffee—and that was a problem. Gum I can go without; coffee I cannot. I have no clue how I functioned without my daily iced nonfat Grande Caramel Macchiato (expensive, yes, but still cheaper than a pregnancy test) while pregnant. Besides the hormones, that's probably one of the main reasons I was so moody all the time. Luckily, as soon as I had my baby, my love for that $4.75 crack in a cup returned.

Other foods that were on my do-not-ingest list: eggs, most fruits but especially bananas, milk—pretty much anything that was healthy and probably beneficial to my body. Good thing for prenatal vitamins. (Side note: Prenatal vitamins have a peculiar taste and are the size of horse pills, which makes them very hard to swallow. They also magically make your pee smell while turning it an awesome shade of fluorescent yellow. Good times!)

(The Baby Bump)

It will take quite a while for your baby bump to appear, especially if this is your first child. Mine didn't show up until around month five. Up until then, I would go out of my way to tell people I was pregnant, just so they wouldn't think I had overdone it on the pie during the holidays. I remember standing in the mirror my first few months of pregnancy convinced I was seeing signs of a bump, when all I was doing was leaning back and pushing my stomach out. (You've probably seen something like this on Facebook before. The pregnant belly selfie is hard to resist.)

Eight months later in the holy-cow-get-this-baby-out-of-me stage, as I stood in front of the same mirror, unable to see my feet, I would regret wishing for a bump so early on.

Once your bump does arrive, you are all of a sudden upgraded to first-class citizenship. People go out of their way to be nice to you. They hold the door, give up their seat, and offer to carry anything you are holding. In some places you even get special parking privileges.

Now that those days are behind me, I often fantasize about walking around with a fake baby belly just so I can feel special again. My advice is, enjoy it while you can, and to absolutely take advantage of the perks. When the bump goes away and you realize that none of your clothes fit anymore and your stomach is just a blob of extra skin, you'll miss that little basketball.

There is one downside of the baby belly worth noting: For some reason, people are drawn to baby bumps like they're magnets. As if in a trance, they will reach out and place their hands directly on your stomach, only to later pull back and then ask your permission. It's weird.

When your bump makes its appearance, decide right away if you are going to be okay with the whole strangers-touching-your-belly thing. For myself, I invoked the grandparent clause. If the person looked like they were old enough to be a grandparent, I gave them the satisfaction of a belly rub—but I (strongly) encouraged everyone else to keep their hands to themselves.

If you don't like the idea of a stranger touching your

bulging belly, try keeping a safe distance between yourself and others at all times while in the late stages of your
pregnancy—and you might want to think about getting a
Taser, too.

(A Whole New Wardrobe)

As your stomach continues to grow, you'll notice something concerning: your clothes no longer fit. This means it's time to spend some money on maternity clothes—but wait! Do not try to buy for yourself in the super early stages of pregnancy. Although those size-small skinny maternity jeans look great in month two, they won't even be able to get up past your ankles by month six. My advice: wait until you have some actual belly to cover up before going on a maternity-wear shopping spree.

The great thing about today's maternity clothes is they are very fashionable. Gone are the days where being pregnant meant getting stuck wearing muumuus for months. But there's a downside to this, of course: fashionable maternity clothes are really freaking expensive, especially considering the fact that you will only be able to wear them for about five months.

Now that I don't have a baby inside me, I realize how ridiculous it is that I have ten pairs of $80 maternity pants in my closet that I will never wear again. (Knock on wood.) But at the time, when I realized how comfortable it was to wear jeans that don't require buttoning and look cute with pretty much any baby bump shirt, I went a little crazy. I call this disease "Maternity Clothes Overindulgence" (MCO), but luckily there are a handful of things you can do to avoid falling victim to it like I did.

Ways to avoid MCO:

1. Take your significant other with you when you go shopping. When they see how much you are about to pay for a maternity tank top, they will escort you out of the store posthaste.

2. Find bargain stores or look for deals online. Some of your cheaper retail stores have great maternity selections. The quality may not be as great as that of the high-end merchandise, but remember, unless you're planning on birthing your very own

Brady Bunch, you won't be wearing these clothes for very long.

3. Some consignment shops and thrift stores have maternity wear, and they can be great sources of barely used and surprisingly stylish attire.

4. Sharing is caring. Odds are you know *someone* who's had kids in the past year or two. See if any of them have something they can pass along to you—and then save your own clothes and pass them on to someone you know when you're done with them.

(Sex? Yes Please)

When I first became pregnant, I was very concerned about having sex. In my mind, with how things work and what goes where, we would surely end up giving my son a black eye.

This, of course, is not true. Unless your doctor has told you to refrain from doing it for some reason, intercourse while pregnant is perfectly safe and will not harm your baby. Even a record-setting-sized dong, dildo, or any other apparatus used for penetration will not come close enough to your bundle of joy to do any damage—at least, that's what my doctor told me.

After hearing this news early on in my pregnancy, I felt reassured—but my husband and I still didn't have very much sexual contact in those first few months. I was just too damn tired all the time. It wasn't until the gift of Holy Trinity Phase Two—"Holy crap, I feel great!"—that I was able to indulge again. The transformation was incredible: as if by magic, I reached month five and my energy level skyrocketed (and conveniently, so did my libido).

My husband was clued into the return of my sexual prowess right away. Normally at the end of the night, we would lie on the couch together, and I would promptly pass out on him. This time, I pounced on him instead.

Sex in the late stages of pregnancy can feel amazing. You experience increased blood flow to your genitals, which can in turn increase the sensation of intercourse. It's also good exercise, so if you are still feeling the prenatal blues at this point in your pregnancy, increasing your endorphins through physical contact is healthy for both your body and your relationship.

There is one major issue to contend with when having sex toward the end of your nine months, and that is navigating around the baby bump. There are only a few positions available, all of which come with some adjustments for comfort. We tried doing it standing up; and we tried doing it with me lying on my side; but ultimately, we found straight-up missionary to be the best option, as it was the most comfortable for me.

If your partner gets anxious about looking at your large baby bump while you're having sex, just tell them to knock it off, close their eyes, and keep going.

(You Are Probably Nesting If . . .)

- You get the urge to clean all of your bathrooms at 1:00 A.M.

- You have folded, unfolded, and refolded all of your new baby clothes for the third time.

- You go into a rage at the sight of the single unwashed dish your partner left in the sink.

- You feel the need to go out and buy bunk beds just in case your baby turns four overnight.

- You find yourself alphabetizing the food in your refrigerator. (Just kidding; this one actually means you have OCD. Seek help!)

I don't remember feeling the need to nest with Baby #1. With Baby #2, though, that instinct was in full effect. Right around the six-month mark, I became an obsessive neat freak. I could not go to bed at night unless the entire house was spotless. My body literally refused to relax until our home looked neat and organized.

For those with toddlers at home you know that keeping your house tidy is close to impossible. No matter how much you try to keep up with the mess during the day, dishes, clothes, and toys just continue to multiply.

In the early stages of my extreme nesting, my husband—seeing my nightly exhaustion and hyperaware of the size of my growing belly—would try to get me to relax and lie down. "Just wait until tomorrow," he'd say. "We can clean it up then." His efforts, of course, were fruitless—enter Ms. Hyde from stage right. Instead of listening to reason, I responded with tears or wrath and continued my cleaning. He soon learned to either help out or get out.

Another memory of nesting I have is when we moved out of our town home and into an actual house. (The town home's living room had been doubling as a toy room for quite some time, so we needed the space.)

The new house was the perfect size for us, but the interior decorations were straight out of the early '90s—gold fixtures everywhere, cream paint throughout, and a massive fluorescent light over the kitchen island. You know, just like the kind you would find in your grade school classroom. For these and other reasons, from the moment we moved into our new home, I had an insatiable urge to have everything redecorated in time for the baby.

My husband thought I was nuts and again tried to get me to slow down. But I couldn't. In my mind, terrible things would happen if the entire house wasn't painted and furnished before I gave birth to baby number two. I was on a mission. And you would be amazed at the willpower of a nesting pregnant woman. I felt like Superwoman. By the time I came home from the hospital, every room had been painted and decorated, the gold was gone, and the fluorescent light was in the trash—all completed while very pregnant, working full time, and raising a toddler.

If you are looking for a decorator, consider looking for one who's expecting; I guarantee she'll work wonders.

(I Gotta Go)

Peeing. Ugh.

The need to pee constantly is something that starts early and only gets worse the more pregnant you become. As your baby grows, he or she puts an increasing amount of weight on your bladder making it harder and harder to "hold it"—which means that for months you will be forced to relieve yourself at all hours of the day and night. It's a huge pain in the ass.

I was up to double-digit pees per day by the end of both my pregnancies. Nights were even worse for me, though; I felt like I was caught up in a vicious cycle of dry mouth and urination. I would down a glass of water before bed, then wake up not too long after needing to go pee, after which I would feel dehydrated again, which meant I would drink more water before heading back to bed, only to wake up an hour later having to go pee again.

This continued every night until I went into labor. Maybe it's nature's sick way of getting you prepared for the sleepless nights that come once your child is born, I don't know. Whatever the reason, our household toilet paper consumption skyrocketed during the forty weeks I was pregnant.

One story I will share—and this goes out to all the ladies who peed on their hands while taking a pregnancy test; hopefully it will make you feel a little better—is about the worst time I had to pee:

I was on my way home from work in Washington, DC, and I got stuck in some major traffic: I was completely stopped at rush hour on 95 south. (If you live in the Beltway, you know how bad it can get there.) I had made sure to pee before leaving my last meeting, but I was toward the end of my pregnancy, and at this point even that kind of foresight only bought me thirty minutes tops.

I hadn't been sitting in traffic for long before I realized I had to go. After trying to ignore it as best I could, I looked around for a cup or any type of container that could aid in my dilemma. There was none to be found. With no exit in sight and no remaining bladder control to speak of, I had only one option: I was going to have to pee my pants.

To save as much face as possible, I grabbed a dry cleaning bag from the backseat and a pair of sweatpants from my suitcase and shoved them both under my butt. I then dropped my pants—and let it go. It was the first time in my life that I had felt intense relief and shame all at the same time. But it's not like I had much of a choice in the matter. It was embarrassing, sure, but it was necessary.

If you ever find yourself in a similar situation during your pregnancy, I hope this story makes you feel better. (And if you were one of the truck drivers who happened to be driving by when all this was taking place and you caught me with my pants down— I hope you enjoyed the free show!)

(An Emotional Mess)

Tears, like night sweats, are an early tip that you may be pregnant. A friend I know who had three children and no plans for another was running a 10K for charity once when, around mile three, she started to well up out of nowhere.

"I was running at a good pace and feeling great," my friend told me. "Then I began to read the backs of the runners' T-shirts in front of me. The sayings were very positive and uplifting, but reading them made me start to cry hysterically."

Since she had already gone through three pregnancies, the sudden tears were an instant giveaway that something was amiss. After her husband picked her up from the finish line, they went straight to the pharmacy—and when they got home, they found out she was indeed pregnant again.

It's not just during the early stages of pregnancy that you'll find yourself weeping uncontrollably, however. As I've already mentioned, your emotions get completely out of control when you're pregnant—and that often means tons of waterworks. The littlest thing can bring you to tears. For me, it was watching TLC's *A Baby Story* while getting dressed in the morning. The second that kid came out on the TV, I would start to cry.

I once asked my husband how he remembered me acting while I was pregnant, and his immediate response was, "You pretty much cried every day." So no, I'm not exaggerating.

There's no real remedy for this issue, but there are a few things you can do to make the tears a bit more manageable: 1) try to carry tissues at all times; 2) avoid the Lifetime channel like the plague; and 3) stay the hell away from any public service announcements staring Sarah McLaughlin.

(Am I Going Through Puberty Again?)

If you were formerly an A cup, those boobs you've wanted your whole life will finally show up when you get pregnant. Your body has to make room for all of the milk you are going to produce, and that means you receive the wonderful gift of natural breast implants.

Looking back on that Halloween night when I was dressed as a sluttier version of Donatello, I remember now that my husband mentioned I was looking a bit bustier than usual. At the time I just figured it was the cheap green plastic material playing mind tricks on him, but now I know the truth: I was pregnant, and my size A's weren't cutting it anymore, so my body was adjusting.

I would have been happy with a full C, but my body didn't stop there; no, the universe thought it would be funny to hit me with a set of E's. Yes, that's right—E's! My boobs got so big I felt like they were the only things people would look at. I had to buy all new bras, went from running to walking for fear of self-incurred black eyes, and was subjected to a flood of new nicknames invented by my friends—"Jugs," "Boobs McGee," and "Torpedoes," to cite just a few.

I had always longed for bigger breasts, but those bad boys were a bit out of control. They were big enough that I'm pretty sure they scared my husband—a *man* afraid of *boobs*? (I wouldn't believe it if I hadn't seen it myself either—but it's a good thing they freaked him out, honestly, because they hurt so badly I wouldn't have let him touch them even if he wanted to.)

I wish I could tell you that after you give birth and are done breastfeeding, your new boobs will stay nice and firm and beautiful. But I would be lying to you.

Immediately after I stopped breastfeeding, my breasts began to reverse in size. After about nine months, (the time it took for them to grow), they were completely deflated. Today they look and feel like two Ziploc bags half full of pudding, and when I lie down at night, I have to pull them out of my out of my armpits and wrestle them back into their rightful place on my chest before falling asleep. Sexy, right?

(Nipples or China?)

Every month that passed while I was pregnant seemed to spark a new bodily change. One such modification—one that I could not help but notice—was the dramatic change of the size and color of my nipples. The further into my pregnancy I progressed, the larger my areolae grew and the darker they became, until one day I looked down and there was a massive pair of brown, dinner-plate-sized nipples staring back at me.

Since my circle of friends was already referring to me as Torpedoes, and because all my former modesty was at this point gone due to the many trips I'd made to the gynecologist throughout my pregnancy, I thought I might as well let everyone in on this curiosity. So one night, when my girlfriends and I were just hanging out at my house, and they were drinking wine and I was jealous, I flashed them the china. It was a full-on National Geographic party in my living room. They were as weirded out as I was. We immediately took to Google to find out what was going on.

It turns out nature knows what it's doing: according to my sources, your nipples naturally grow and darken in color during pregnancy so that by the time your baby comes out and you want to nurse him or her, it's not too hard for the little one to find them and latch on. Not that awesome to look at, I'll admit, but a very cool idea from Mother Nature nonetheless.

(Stretch Marks and Varicose Veins, Oh My!)

Boo to stretch marks! Those pesky lines seem to show up out of nowhere, and if you are not one of the lucky ones, they stay for life. They say that cocoa butter helps, but I had a hard enough time remembering to take my prenatal vitamins, let alone lather up on a daily basis. Maybe I should have tried harder, though, because to this day I have lines down my side—not my favorite part of my post-baby body.

Another gnarly set of lines that can appear during and after pregnancy are varicose veins. As your body continues to grow and swell, the pressure put on your veins causes them to increase in size. The result: large blue and red lines found just under the surface of your skin for all to see. This visually unappealing pregnancy symptom is often hereditary, but there are some things you can do to prevent them from coming.

First off, the heavier you are the greater your chances of developing varicose veins, so exercise and healthy eating habits are a good way to protect yourself. To reduce swelling in your legs—the area of your body most prone to varicose veins—try not to sit or stand for long periods of time, and when you do sit, keep your legs uncrossed if you can. A final measure you can take is to wear compression socks. They are not very fashionable, but they are temporary, unlike the even less stylish "veiny" look you may end up with if you don't wear them.

Both my mother and sister gained permanent black-and-blue squiggles on their thighs and calves during and following their pregnancies, so I was sure I was headed for varicose town as well when I got knocked up. But somehow I lucked out and avoided swelling of the veins altogether.

If you aren't one of the lucky ones and you end up developing varicose veins, there is a good chance they will go away on their own after the birth of your baby. If they don't, there are a number of cure-alls out there. If it comes to that, consult your doctor first!

(Butt Buttons)

And then there are hemorrhoids. Ugh. I always thought hemorrhoids were something only men got from spending too much time on the porcelain throne, but I learned just how wrong I was during my first pregnancy. Turns out they're common in women as well, especially pregnant women. Lucky us, right?

Hemorrhoids aren't harmful, but that doesn't make them any less unpleasant. Common or not, I was not very enthused the first time I went to wipe and found a little bump that didn't belong. I had enough going on down there as it was. What was this curious (and possibly concerning) addition?

I immediately went to see my doctor, who confirmed that my mystery bump was, in fact, a hemorrhoid. Yuck. I don't know why, but I am just bothered by the word "hemorrhoid." It sounds so, so awful—more awful than the actual condition it refers to, in my opinion. I think we should change the name to make it sound less horrifying. How about "butt button"? (Is that any less gross? I think so, but you'll have to decide for yourself.)

Anyway, my butt button hung out all through both of my pregnancies. There are creams and various wipes available for the irritation that causes butt buttons, but nothing I found would make that sucker go away.

My button decreased in size after each of my kids were born, but it's never fully gone away, and every once and a while it makes a comeback. On a recent girl's trip, for example, I laughed so hard that I giggled the sucker right back out! I've been told you can have surgery to remove butt buttons, but the thought of undergoing a procedure like that is more disturbing to me than the word hemorrhoid, so I've decided to simply make my peace with my button and leave things be.

Side note: *Hemorrhoids—I mean, butt buttons—are no big deal. But if yours starts to itch or burn, or doesn't decrease in size after the birth of your child, you should definitely consult a doctor!*

Oh Where, Oh Where Did My Belly Button Go?

It's like watching grass grow—you don't notice it on a daily basis, but at the end of every month, your belly button slowly disappears just a little bit more. By the end of my pregnancy, my innie was an outie. Nature's cooking thermometer, letting me know my turkey was done.

If you're especially attached to your innie, don't worry: you'll get yours back after you have your baby, though it will probably be a lot bigger than it used to be.

(Cankles)

I booed stretch marks; I am going to double boo cankles. At the end of pregnancy you don't look or feel as cute as you did when your baby bump first arrived for a number of reasons, and cankles (when your ankles are the same size as your calves) are one of my least favorite additions to the list.

Both of my kids were born in the summer, and since it was more comfortable to wear dresses than pants, I was forced to flaunt my giant ankles in the warmer months leading up to their births. I looked—and I'm not exaggerating—like a circus tent propped up by a pair of tree stumps.

Side note: Some cankle action is normal, but keep an eye on those bad boys. If the swelling seems to worsen or doesn't go away, consult your doctor.

(Superhuman Scent)

Have you ever had a discussion with your friends about what kind of superpower you would choose if you had to pick just one? Was yours the ability to fly, X-ray vision, or Spidey-sense? Well, I am happy to announce that pregnancy comes with a superpower of its own: a superhuman sense of smell.

I can only assume that this heightened olfactory ability goes back to our animalistic instinct to smell out predators as a way to protect our young—but no matter what the reason, it is pretty cool. My entire pregnancy, I could smell almost anything and instantly know what that smell was—popcorn, hamburgers on the grill, coffee, and once even Teen Spirit deodorant (a throwback to middle school).

Clearly this particular superpower can be good or bad, depending on the scent. The worst experience I can remember was the time I was speaking in front of a group about the stock market and my supernose keyed in on a man sitting in the front row. He must have woken up that morning, poured an entire bottle of cologne into the bathtub, and then hopped in after it.

I tried to remain focused on my talking points, but every time I took a breath, my nostrils felt like they were going to burn off. By the end of my presentation, I had tears in my eyes and my stomach was doing cartwheels.

I hurried out of the room, my tree trunks moving as fast as possible, and ran to the bathroom, where I promptly vomited in the sink.

All that just because some idiot overdid it on the cologne. Superpowers aren't always what they're cracked up to be.

(Who Wrote on My Belly?)

At some point during your pregnancy, you may wake up to find a dark line running down your stomach all the way to your hoo-ha (scientifically called the linea nigra).

In my case, I literally woke up one morning and it was just magically there. It was kind of like the time in college when I fell asleep (passed out) at a party and when I woke up, all sorts of lines and graphics had mysteriously appeared on my body. Although mostly illegible, I was able to make out a number of phallus-like figures. This of course had nothing to do with a natural, pregnancy-related occurrence and everything to do with my jerk friends. The best part? They had attacked me with a *permanent* marker. It took me hours to wash off all of the dicks and smiley faces.

Waking up to find penises all over your body is not normal and probably a good "drink in moderation" alert. Waking up to find a linea nigra on your stomach, however, is an entirely natural thing, and very normal. Your hormones play a role in creating it, and while I'm pretty sure it doesn't do anything to help with pregnancy or your baby, it's also not permanent. It'll last through your pregnancy and for a little while beyond it, but it should fade away a few months after you give birth.

(The Great Teeth-Brushing Massacre)

I consider myself to have pretty decent dental hygiene. I brush my teeth twice a day and floss on holidays. But when I was pregnant, I spit into the sink after brushing one evening and looked down to find a massive amount of blood staring back at me.

Startled, I looked up into the mirror and smiled wide to inspect the damage—and my teeth and gums were so red, it looked like I had been punched in the mouth.

Apparently excess blood pools in your gums when you become pregnant. Fun, right?

But surprisingly, gross as spitting blood into the sink every night was, having bloody gums came in handy for me at one point:

I was six months pregnant when it came time for me to go to the dentist for a cleaning. I am one of those people who, no matter how hard I try, can never remember to floss. Brush twice a day, no problem—but add those few extra minutes to floss? Not a chance. The idea just doesn't even cross my mind.

As a result, every time I go to the dentist I end up having to sit and listen to a lecture on the atrocities of gingivitis and why flossing is the next best thing since sliced bread. So when I got my reminder in the mail, I felt that familiar sinking sensation. *Ugh. Here we go again.*

But then I had a light bulb moment: *On this trip in,* I realized, *my gums are going to bleed no matter what. They'll have no clue if I've been abiding by their stupid flossing rules or not!*

Suddenly, a trip to the dentist didn't sound so onerous. The day of my appointment, I sat cheerful in the chair as I bled all over the place. The dentist said not to worry the gum bleeding was due to my pregnancy. Phew, shame averted! When I was done I walked out of there head held high, feeling like I'd finally beaten the dental system.

Expect to witness a Friday the 13th–like massacre in your sink bowl twice a day throughout your forty weeks. But like so many other weird things that happen to your body during pregnancy, the phenomenon should only last until your baby is born; after that, your gums will go back to normal. If they don't, you should probably get that checked out—though if you're a delinquent flosser like me, you may want to wait until your next cleaning to do it. (Kidding, kidding. Get that taken care of!)

(Alien in My Belly)

One of the things I was looking forward to the
most about being pregnant was feeling my baby kick. Actually, it wasn't so much that I needed to feel *my* baby do it—I
really just wanted to feel *a* baby do it. But since I would
never dare touch another person's pregnant belly (for fear
of being tased), I knew I would have to wait until I was the
pregnant one to cross that experience off my bucket list.

I was right around twenty weeks pregnant, lying in
bed, when I felt the first flutter.

Me: "I think I just felt the baby kick."
Husband: "Really?"

Then, sure enough, there was that feeling again—a very faint movement coming from my belly.

Me: "Yes, I just felt it again."
Husband: "Cool, let me feel!"

Of course as soon as my husband put his hand to my stomach, all motion ceased. This game of baby kicking cat and mouse persisted throughout the remainder of the night and he went to bed without getting the chance to feel our baby kick. The next day my husband told me he thought I was making the whole thing up. When he was finally able to feel the baby kicking for himself a few nights later, he recanted his former accusation.

As time went on the kicks became more frequent, but the excitement of feeling them never seemed to go away. Every time I felt something, in fact, I had to announce it to my husband. Looking back, I can see how annoying this must have been for him. Especially since the baby moved almost exclusively at night, you know, while my husband was either asleep or trying to get there.

Me: "He kicked again."
Husband: "Shhh."
Me: "Kick . . . kick . . . another!"
Husband: "Shhh."
Me: "He is moving a lot."

Husband: *No response.*
Me: "Good one."
Husband: *No response.*
Me: "Kick."
Husband: "Go to sleep."
Me: "Okay, good night . . . kick!"

You get the point.

While your child has been doing water aerobics for months by this point, you probably won't notice it happening until the end of the second trimester. It will start out as a soft tap—but at the end of pregnancy, when your baby has reached its final fruit size (watermelon, if you're interested), that tap-like kick will have been replaced by full-blown somersaults. In your final trimester, there will be times when you will be able to look down and see the outline of an entire hand or foot pressed against your stomach. Very cool and yet gross at the same time—kind of like the epic "chestburster" scene in *Alien*.

When Did I Become a Member of the Golden Girls?

As my pregnancy progressed I started to undergo a number of system and body malfunctions I had always associated with old age. Turns out that being pregnant is not so different from growing decrepit. Some symptoms they have in common include:

1. **Frequent urination:** I never actually dove all the way into my old lady role and resorted to wearing Depends, but looking back on it, maybe I should have—I could have saved a good pair of sweatpants.

2. **Hot flashes:** Like an aging woman, a pregnant woman goes through lots of hormonal changes. One minute you are freezing. The next you're overheating. My husband would get so mad at me at night because I would steal all of the covers when I was cold, and then whip them back at him when I got too hot. Somehow, our marriage survived this.

3. **Swelling of the hands and feet:** This can increase during the summer months and especially toward the end of pregnancy. During both of my pregnancies, I had to stop wearing high heels because I could no longer get them on my feet. At least, that's what I told myself. It's also possible that I stopped wearing them because I had gained so much weight I was afraid I'd snap a heel if I even tried.

4. **Carpal tunnel:** This was the worst and one of the more shocking things that happened while I was pregnant. In my last trimester during both of my pregnancies, I began to get shooting pain in my hands and arms. At one point it got so bad that I would lie awake at night with my arms dangling off the side of the bed, hoping against hope that if I could just find the right position, the pain would stop. A visit to the doctor confirmed that I had pregnancy-induced carpal tunnel. Which, appar-

ently, is pretty common and happens when your pregnancy-related swelling puts pressure on the nerves in your hands and arms. After my children were born, I had to get cortisone shots, as well as take an anti-inflammatory medication, to get the pain to subside.

5. **Heartburn:** Changes in hormones during pregnancy can cause the muscles in the esophagus to relax, which then allows stomach acid to rise up. (I looked that up on the Internet.) And I was a glutton for punishment when it came to heartburn during my pregnancy, because I wasn't willing to give up one of my favorite foods: Thai, cooked medium spicy (which for an American tongue, as you probably know, means *hot*). Even though I knew it would lead to heartburn—even though I knew how uncomfortable I would be afterward—I ate Thai food weekly while I was pregnant. This meant that I suffered from bad heartburn at least once a week until my baby was born. It sucked. But coconut milk can be so addictive!

6. **Hair growth:** I assume it was due to the prenatal vitamins, but while pregnant I had an amazing head of hair. It rocked. I would have made a great Vidal Sassoon model. Unfortunately, my head was not the

only area where I experienced an increase in follicle growth. It also happened in some not so amazing places, like my upper lip, nipples, and happy trail. I'm proud to say that I kept up with my increased need for lady landscaping (you know what I'm talking about) until I was about seven months along. At that point, however, I could barely see my feet, let alone my bathing suit line, so instead of risking my crotch's life, I went au naturel after that until I gave birth. Bringing back that eighties bush!!

7. **Hair loss:** The Lord giveth and the Lord taketh away. Just as I was getting used to my newly luscious locks, I gave birth and it was like someone hit an off switch connected directly to my scalp. In the months that followed, I began to experience hair loss and not just any hair loss, *rapid* hair loss. Every time I took a shower, clumps of hair fell out. It was frightening. We had to get a plumber to unclog our shower drain because of it. The molting seems to have subsided now, but I don't think my hair will ever look as good as it did pre-delivery again.

8. **Fatigue:** This is something that can be different for everyone. Some women experience sporadic bouts of exhaustion; others are pretty much tired throughout their entire pregnancy. For me, fatigue barbelled

both of my pregnancies: I was tired in the first three months and tired in the last three months. I looked forward to being done with that feeling toward the end of my first pregnancy, blissfully unaware of how much *more* exhausted I would be once the baby arrived. That was a fun post-pregnancy discovery.

9. **Back pain:** Obviously, the larger you become, the more stress your body—specifically, your back—has to endure. And those torpedo boobs don't help. You may want to invest in a heating pad.

10. **Memory loss:** People joke about "pregnancy brain," but I'm here to tell you that it is a real thing. While you're pregnant, you may find yourself completely forgetting what you are doing or where you've put things on a regular basis. I resorted to creating lists and e-mailing myself tasks throughout the day so I wouldn't forget. That helped when it came to most things. Unfortunately, I had no way of e-mailing myself in advance of losing my keys, something that happened at least once every other week. It helps to have a sense of humor about your memory missteps; or, alternatively, you can duct tape your personal belongings to yourself to ensure that you'll be able to find them at all times.

11. **Flatulence and constipation:** Hormones slow digestion, often leading to excess gas and constipation. Exercise can help minimize these symptoms, as it helps increase motility in the gastrointestinal tract. Avoiding broccoli, beans, dried fruit, and carbonated drinks can help too. But no matter what you do, you'll probably experience both of these things more than once during pregnancy. It comes with the territory; get used to it.

12. **Insomnia:** In the beginning of pregnancy, all you will want to do is close your eyes and fall asleep, and you'll be pleasantly surprised by how easy that will be to do. In my first trimester, all I had to do was sit down and shut my eyes, and I would be out like a light within seconds. But all this changes at the end of pregnancy.

In the "holy cow, get this baby out of me stage," you have multiple forces working against you:

1. Your stomach is so large you can't get comfortable.

2. If by some miracle you do manage to get comfortable, you'll have to get up and pee in two minutes, ruining everything.

3. Your mind is a frenzy of nesting concerns.

4. You have stomach acid in your throat because you insisted on eating Thai food again.

5. You're probably in the process of sweating through yet another pair of pajamas.

At this point, just like when I had to force myself to nap, I resorted to YouTube "Sleep Meditation" videos to get some shut-eye. They were very helpful in calming my scattered brain, as well as getting my body to relax. It only took a few minutes of listening before the voices lulled me to sleep. But I'm going to give it to you straight: Even the best meditation videos are no match for a watermelon on your bladder. At this point, sleeping through the entire night—ever—is highly unlikely.

(The Baby Registry)

Somewhere around month five of your pregnancy— usually after you find out what sex your baby is going to be (if you decide to do this)—it is time to plan a baby shower. And the first thing you will be encouraged to do to prepare for this event is create a list of things you will need when your baby arrives.

Creating a baby registry sounds simple in theory, I know. But how are you supposed to know what you're going to need for your baby if you've never had one before?

The first time my husband and I walked into the baby megastore that shall not be named to create our registry, they handed us something that looked like a gun and a giant list of things we would "need" and said, "Start shopping." We took two steps forward, stared at the never-ending aisles of baby supplies for a minute or so, and promptly turned around and walked out. When we were safely outside those glass sliding doors, my husband announced, "I think I need a drink." As I was sure I had cried, yelled, or silent-treated him at least once that day already, I was happy to step in as his post–baby registry debacle designated driver.

To say we were completely overwhelmed would be an understatement. How were we supposed to know what to get? Not only were there thousands of items, there were duplicates of those items. Which brand was the best? We had zero experience with babies. We were not prepared.

When we got home, we decided to call everyone we knew with kids to find out exactly what we would and would not need. And it was great: the next time we ventured into the store to complete our registry, we were armed with some solid information, and managed to put about fifty items on our list in record time.

"Here it is," I said when we were done, proudly handing our list to the store clerk.

"That's it?" she asked. "Most people have around 150 items on their list."

"That's because most people get ripped off by you guys," I shot back.

Okay, I didn't actually say that—even though it's definitely true. Instead, I said something like, "Well, we can always come back if we find we need something else."

Below is a list of items I have been sharing with all of my pregnant friends. I hope it will be helpful to you as well:

MUST-HAVES

Day-to-Day Items:

- **Diapers in various sizes:** Our two-year-old is now in size six, and our three-week-old is still in newborn diapers. You will spend a ton of money on diapers while raising your child, so stock up while you can. We ended up using most of our gift cards for diaper purchases. If you are one of the daring, environmentally conscious people going the reusable diaper route, I commend you. Happy cleaning.

- **Wipes:** Just like diapers, you will go through tons of wipes. Stock up.

- **Butt cream:** Babies poop daily and their little bums are always red.

- **Baby lotion:** Newborn skin gets very dry.

- **Baby shampoo:** Tear-Free Shampoo and Wash.

- **Blankets:** I find you can't have too many blankets. You will be putting your baby down all over the house, so you will want to have blankets ready to go in each room.

- **Burp cloths:** These are essential—unless, of course, you don't mind ruining all your clothes, in which case, feel free to forego these.

- **Crib sheets and plastic mattress pad:** It is still a mystery to me how tiny babies with bladders the size of a bean can pee through their diaper and their clothes, but it happens.

- **Nail kit:** I was scared to death the first time we cut our first baby's nails, but it had to be done. Those suckers get sharp.

- **Baby mittens:** Put these on your baby's hands until you get enough guts to clip their nails.

- **First-aid kit:** We keep one in the house and one in the car.

- **Thermometer:** We got one for the butt (sorry little ones), and one for the ear. They have ones for the foreheads as well, but I am not convinced those are as accurate.

- **Baby monitor:** If you can afford it, go with the video monitor. You can actually see what your child is doing, which is a huge relief, since when they're really little you're convinced that they're going to stop breathing any second.

- **Books:** This is the only "toy" I recommend registering for. You can never have too many books.

Feeding Supplies:

- **Breast pump:** If you will be breast-feeding, you'll need a pump.

- **Milk storage set:** This can be found in the same aisle with the breast pumps, and is necessary if you're pumping.

- **Bottles:** Get size one nipples. You can get bigger ones later, as your child grows.

- **Bottle rack:** This is great for organization.

- **Bottle brush:** You will use this multiple times a day, every day.

- **Bibs:** Avoid infant size and go for one size fits all. You will be using these for a long time.

- **Child-sized bowls, plates, and utensils:** You won't need these right away, but you may as well have someone else buy them for you.

Items for You:

***You do not have to put these on your registry if you find it too embarrassing, but YOU WILL NEED them.*

- **Nipple cream:** Dry, cracked nipples are painful and pretty much impossible to avoid if you're breast-feeding.

- **Breast-feeding bras:** These make it easier to feed your child without having to totally disrobe.

- **Breast pads:** These prevent you from walking around with two wet dots on display. When your milk comes in, your nipples will leak a lot, breast pads help to absorb those leaks and prevent you from walking around with two wet dots on display.

- **Big underwear:** There is a lot going on down there after you have a baby, so you will want full coverage.

- **Pads:** You may bleed for weeks after having the baby . . . brutal.

Big Items:

- **Crib:** We got the kind that converts to a bed, but we didn't end up using the bed.

- **Mattress:** My husband thought, "the softer the better," but the opposite is actually true. Get something firm for your baby!

- **Changing table:** Although your couch or floor will work, changing tables keep you from hunching over, which can help your back. They also usually come with extra storage—and believe me, you'll need that.

- **Rocker:** Our first child had colic, so we spent hours rocking back and forth.

- **Car seat:** It may make sense to get a car seat/ stroller combo, but either way, you obviously need one of these to keep your baby safe in the car! They also won't let you leave the hospital without one.

- **Stroller:** I prefer strollers with rubber wheels, because they are more durable. But no matter what type of stroller you go with, test it out in advance. We bought a jogging stroller, and the first time I attempted a pace faster than a walk the wheels shook so badly I had to slow down immediately. Exercising is important, but not as important as preventing your baby from getting shaken-baby syndrome.

- **Umbrella stroller:** This is a smaller stroller that folds up easily and is great for travel, especially if you plan on flying with your child.

Miscellaneous:

- **Baby seat or bouncer:** You need a place (besides a crib) where you can safely put your baby down.

- **Baby carrier:** This is a great, hands-free way to tote your child around, and an essential piece of equipment if you have multiple children.

- **Mobile for the crib:** To this day, our two-year-old loves his mobile.

- **Baby activity seat:** These are great for early learning, and to give your arms a break.

ITEMS YOU MAY WANT TO WAIT ON BUYING:

- **Bureau for the nursery:** Only buy one if it fits and you think you will use it for clothes later on. Most changing tables have plenty of room for baby clothes, and if you have a closet you can use that space too.

- **Baby swing:** We spent a ton of money on the latest and greatest swing, only to find out that both of our children hated it.

- **Formula:** If you're not breastfeeding, you'll want to wait to find out which formula your baby can tolerate before stocking up.

- **Baby bath:** We found the sink was easier than a baby bath; you might want to try out your own sink before investing in a bath.

- **High chair:** You won't need this until they are able to sit on their own. We got the one that attaches to a normal chair to reserve space. Warning: with the food remnants and overall wear and tear, we did end up destroying the chair

- **Pacifiers:** Some babies like them and some don't. They will give you some at the hospital to try out.

- **Cloth to put over your shopping cart:** We got one and never used it.

- **Mirror to hang on your backseat to see your baby:** Again, we got one and never used it.

- **Pack 'n Play:** If you plan on traveling or want a second place for your baby to nap this will come in handy.

- **Diaper pail:** We bought the latest and greatest model, and the changing area still stank. You may as well save your money and just get a regular trashcan with regular trash bags. It's a losing battle.

- **Baby gate:** Get one if you have stairs, but otherwise, you probably don't need it.

- **Walker:** Our son could never figure out how to go forward and ended up stuck and upset. Total fail.

DO NOT REGISTER FOR . . .

- **Baby Clothes:** You will get tons. We still have items with tags on them.

- **Toys:** You will get a million of these, many of which will be duplicates.

- **Baby-wipe warmer:** It doesn't work—and even worse, it dries out the wipes!

- **Baby bottle warmer:** Ours worked for a short time then one day it burned the bottom of the bottle, so we chucked it.

(Baby Showers)

I am not a fan of baby showers. No offense if you have been really looking forward to yours, but most of them are incredibly boring and drag on for way too long.

Given how much I had dreaded going to every baby shower I'd ever attended, when it came time to have one of my own, I did whatever I could to make it bearable for my guests—and I think I might have actually succeeded.

Here are some tips if you are in the same camp I am:

1. Have good food and drinks.

2. Serve mimosas if it makes sense.

3. Open your gifts while people are eating, so your guests have something to do and aren't just staring at you for an hour.

4. Open your gifts in a respectful but timely manner. (I have a huge family, and there were probably ninety people at my baby shower. That means lots of presents. Can you imagine how long it would have taken if I had opened every little thing from every person and held it up? Hours.) The best thing to do is give the room a summary of the item(s) and if you see the person who got you the gift, acknowledge them while opening.

5. Have someone keep a record of who got you what gift as you go.

6. Did I mention mimosas?

7. Have attendees fill out self-addressed envelopes before they leave. This will save your hands from going numb when you send out your thank-you cards.

8. Keep the party to a maximum of two hours. If people want to stay longer they can, but don't make anyone feel like they should.

9. Avoid overly crowded or hot locations.

10. If you must have games, keep them quick. (Also, guessing what chocolate bar is melted in the diaper is gross and should be avoided at all cost.)

(The Waiting Game)

By now you have puked, peed, slept, peed, yelled, cried, tossed, turned, peed, grown, nested, and peed some more. Friends and family have showered you with gifts you will never use, you have a few baby names picked out for the final cut, and you are the size of a blimp—but it is still not time to have your baby. Why does it feel like the end of your pregnancy is taking forever? Surprise! Pregnancy is actually longer than nine months!

Let's do the math. It takes forty weeks to grow a baby to full term. On average, there are four weeks in a month. Forty divided by four equals ten, not nine. WTF! Why doesn't anyone tell you that from the get-go? At least then you wouldn't feel so anxious during the last month.

I too just assumed pregnancy would take nine months, because that was the time frame I was used to hearing. I didn't give the matter much thought until I reached the ninth month and it dawned on me that I still had thirty days to go until my technical "due date." Those thirty days were the longest days of my entire pregnancy. Time just seemed to drag on and on, and I began to feel like my baby would never be born.

Welcome to the waiting game. Everyone you talk to toward the end of your pregnancy will say, "Wow, it's gone by so fast," or "Any day now. You are so close." And this will annoy the crap out of you, because you will be larger than ever, and you won't feel like "any day" will ever come. Unlike those other people, you will know that your due date is exactly three weeks, two days, thirteen hours, and twenty-two minutes away, and if you are like me, you will be secretly wishing for your water to break early.

I got so antsy in my final month that I did everything to try and speed the process up. I ate spicy food (heartburn), walked everywhere I could, got pregnancy massages, and upped the intercourse with my husband (finding a comfortable sex position while nine-months pregnant is no easy feat). None of this is scientifically proven to work, however, and of course none of it did.

My only advice to make the waiting game more bearable is to try and fill your time with things you won't be able to do once you are in full-time mommy mode. For example: go to a movie; go out to dinner; go away for the weekend; read a book; have a social life; SLEEP.

Notice that the last word on my list is in capital letters. Take note. If there was one thing many people told me to do before I had my first child, it was sleep, but at the time I didn't fully understand what they meant. Then I gave birth, and suddenly I got it—too late, alas. Let me break it down for you: As an adult, you are used to six to ten hours of uninterrupted sleep a night. But the second you have a newborn, that goes away. Forever. And it's not like your body is magically okay with this sudden change. It hates it. But once you have that baby, all the wishing in the world won't get you more sleep. So instead of wishing the last few weeks of pregnancy away, try sleeping them away instead.

(Packing Your Bags)

My husband and I did a very poor job of packing our bag the first go-round. We only brought one outfit for the baby, a change of clothes for me, and a few toiletries. Not only was this not enough for a normal birth, it certainly didn't cover the extended stay we ended up having in the hospital due to the C-section I underwent.

We had to rely on friends and family to deliver extra sets of clothes for me and the baby, plus books, magazines, and a deck of cards to pass the time. The only other options were trying to find something halfway decent to watch on the fourteen-channel television or walking the halls in a hospital gown and underwear large enough to cover my butt and half of my back. Looking back I am not even sure my husband changed his clothes until a few days into our stint in the hospital. I barely packed anything for the baby and me; I know we didn't pack anything at all for him. Here is a list of items that we should have packed, and that I strongly recommend you have ready to go as you near the end of your pregnancy:

1. **Things to keep you busy.** Magazines, playing cards, crossword puzzles, a good book, computer, phone, and phone charger . . . anything you can think of that will provide entertainment. All they provide you with at the hospital is a television with limited channels, and maybe, if you're lucky, the possibility of overhearing a little gossip from the nurse's station. It gets old fast, trust me.

2. **Snacks.** Have you ever heard that hospitals are known for their cooking? No? Well, there's a reason for that. Bring your own food. You'll thank me later. My husband brought me a fresh sandwich from our favorite deli on my second day in the hospital, and you would have thought he was bringing me a steak dinner.

3. **Camera.** A smart phone will do, but bring *something* to document with! During my second birth,

which was as scheduled C-section, the anesthesiologist actually volunteered to step in as photographer. Although slightly on the graphic side, it is pretty neat to have photos of your child's grand entrance into the world.

4. **Comfy clothes.** Sweatpants, shirts, and socks. You never know how long you'll be there; you might as well be comfortable. And bring them for you and your partner. (I made my husband stay all three nights with me in the hospital when we had our first child. Afterward, I realized that was cruel and unusual punishment. There was no reason for him to be hunched on a small fold-up seat, waking up at all hours of the night, just to sit and stare while I fed the baby. But if you feel the need to torture your significant other as I did, go ahead and pack clothes for them too.)

5. **Large underwear.** You will have a lot of recovering going on down there. Bring multiple pairs of granny panties.

6. **Nursing bras.** Pretty handy if you're nursing.

7. **Toiletries.** The tiny bottles of shampoo and conditioner the hospital provides are not really ade-

quate. Besides, there's not a whole lot that's comfortable about being in the hospital; having your own products with you can help make your stay feel more like home.

8. Two or three newborn outfits for your baby.

Usually babies stay in the clothes the hospital provides until it is time to go home, but some Kodak moments call for a quick change. Come prepared!

(Quiet on the Set . . .)
and Action!

During my pregnancy, I tried to imagine what
delivery day would be like, but my only frame of reference
was what I had seen on television or in the movies. In my
mind, therefore, when the big day came, my water would
break and I would suddenly be in intense pain. My husband and I would then rush, like two crazy people, to the
hospital, and we would immediately deliver a baby.

Here's what really happened:

My water did break and we did slightly panic, but it
took twenty-six hours of labor and a C-section to get that

sucker out. And that is just my story; I have spoken to tons of other women and I can promise you, having a baby is nothing like it's portrayed in the movies.

Here is a list of common movie myths that I feel morally obligated to debunk for you:

1. **Everyone's water breaks.** After watching loads of movies that show women going into labor, I spent my whole life under the assumption that everyone's water breaks. I was shocked to discover the truth, which is that the majority of women's amniotic sacs do not break prior to labor. If you are one of the few, like me, to experience your water breaking, there are a couple of scenarios that can happen: 1) you can have a large gush similar to peeing yourself (which my car and I are very familiar with); 2) you can experience the less intense slow drip, which is harder to identify, especially if you are rocking highly absorbent granny panties. When my water broke during my first pregnancy, I felt the large gush all over my couch and a continued drip all the way to the doctor's office—messy. If your water breaks, I highly recommend carrying a towel with you to the hospital.

2. **Your water breaking leads to turbo-charged contractions.** A second myth I picked up from

the big screen was that having your water break means you will immediately commence excruciatingly painful contractions. Again, not true. Your uterus may start to contract after your amniotic sac breaks, but going straight to level-ten pain is highly unlikely. It is usually a bit more gradual. Oddly, I had *no* contractions after my water broke, so I ended up having to be induced because my cervix wasn't even dilated. Whether you have pain or not, your water breaking is an indication that labor will eventually follow, so call your doctor immediately, and follow his or her instructions.

3. **Labor is fast.** This is the worst. Just because you, Mr. Director, only have five minutes to shoot the labor scene does not mean it is right to mislead viewers into believing that delivering a baby is fast. Labor isn't fast; it lasts *hours.* With your first child, in fact, it's very common to have labor last ten to twenty hours. Yes, you read that correctly—double-digit hours. So be prepared for lots of waiting around time. When my mom found out my water broke early, she panicked. She assumed she was going to miss the birth of her first grandchild. Both she and my mother-in-law paid a hefty price to get on the next flight out

of Boston to Virginia, where we live, then rented a car and sped to the hospital, only to find me twelve hours into labor with no progress at all. They ended up waiting another fourteen hours before our little man entered the world. You're welcome, airline with the free blue potato chips, for the extra $1,800 you received from two caring grandmas-to-be.

4. **All births take place in a hospital.** In the movies, it would be very rare to see a women give birth anywhere other than at an actual hospital. There is the occasional medical drama that will show a women in labor who doesn't make it to the E.R. in time and is then forced to give birth in her car, but she was still on her way to a hospital in the first place. In real life many women create birth plans that do not include a hospital at all. Some prefer to work with a doula instead of a doctor, and end up having their babies at a birthing center or even in their own homes. This is not my cup of tea, as I had my heart set on an immediate epidural upon first hint of pain. However, if it something you are interested in, do some research. In the end you should do what is best for the comfort and safety of you and your baby.

5. **Ten centimeters and the baby is out.** There are many stages of labor. The final stage is the pushing. On film, once the woman's cervix is at ten centimeters, it usually takes thirty to sixty seconds of pushing and then bam, the baby arrives. In real life, this stage of labor can take a while. (Are you seeing a pattern here?) The baby's head and shoulders need to be positioned just right in order to make it out of you. When my sister had her baby, she pushed for four straight hours. At one point the doctor had her on her hands and knees to try and move the baby into the correct position. Finally after a marathon of yoga-like positions, suctioning, an episiotomy (a procedure not for the faint of heart), and the mindset of Superwoman, she got her child out. Thank you, directors, for never showing the true details of a vaginal delivery; because of you, the human race will continue to procreate.

6. **Women do not poop during labor.** Human excrement is not something the rating agencies look on fondly, so the movies disregard it all together. But in reality, most women do poop during labor. You may not know this, but when they tell you to push, they tell you to push exactly like you would when you are trying to take a crap. Knowing that,

it makes sense that during all of that pushing you will certainly push out more than just the baby. Don't be embarrassed. The nurses are used to this, and will get it cleaned up right away.

7. **Delivering a baby is mess-free.** Some movies do show the baby covered in a small amount of gunk, but if you take notice, the mother, the bed, and the hospital floor are clean. Fortunately for viewers, pretty much every director in the history of film has forgotten to account for the fluid, the blood, the poop, and the afterbirth. I know "afterbirth" sounds gross; well, guess what—it is. And it is also the most underestimated part of labor. Following the delivery of your child, you also have to deliver the placenta and fetal membranes. If your partner is squeamish, or if you want to prevent them from having nightmares for life, do not let them witness this part of your delivery. A friend of mine, and father of three put it best: To avoid this happening, he told me, instruct your partner to play "follow the baby." Baby comes out, follow the baby. Baby is handed to mom, follow the baby. Baby is handed to nurse, follow the baby. Nurse takes baby away from mom to be weighed, follow the baby. Afterbirth avoided. It's as simple as that.

8. Babies are always born via the vagina. I know you know this is a myth, but I wish the movies would at least show a few women having cesareans. If they did, it would seem a lot more normal—and maybe I wouldn't have cried when I found out *I* had to have a C-section. When I found out I wasn't going to be able to deliver my baby the "normal" way, I felt like I'd just lost a hugely important battle. I remember breaking into tears and apologizing to my husband that I couldn't get the baby out on my own. He, of course, did not care at all how the baby came out, as long as we were both okay, but at the time I really felt ashamed. Had I known that about one-third of women have cesareans, I would have felt better about it. I would also have been less nervous if I'd known how pain-free and fast the procedure is.

My second time around was much easier. Since I'd had a C-section with my first child and knew what to expect, I elected to go with a scheduled caesarean for my second. And let me tell you, it was a walk in the park. Instead of twenty-six hours of grueling labor—confined to a bed, without access to food or drink—I walked into the operating room, and thirty minutes later they wheeled me out, baby in tow. It was a piece of cake. But I guess that version of labor's just not dramatic enough for the big screen.

9. **You will look like a million bucks once you give birth.** Hollywood likes beautiful people, so therefore it only makes sense that a women in the movie's who has just given birth should look like she has just stepped out of the salon. I promise you no matter how great your stylist is, there is no way you will look movie ready after hours of labor. Even though the producers get the look wrong, I have to give them credit for capturing the reaction of new mom's quite well. When your baby is handed to you for the first time you will cry, smile, and laugh all at the same time. It is truly an amazing feeling. The ordeal you just went through—the pregnancy and the delivery—disappears from memory completely. All you're thinking about now is that little being cradled in your arms. After the birth of our first child, I was overtaken with happiness while in the recovery room. I remember telling my husband in a very perky tone, "Well, that wasn't that bad." He looked at me like I was crazy. "You were just in labor for twenty-six hours, had two epidurals that didn't fully work, were starved and deprived of water for hours, puked your guts out, had your torso cut wide open, and then sewn back up. Not that bad?" Maybe that's why *women* bear the children.

10. Babies come out beautiful. Have you ever noticed how perfect "newborn" babies in the movies look? That is because they are not actual newborns. Actual newborns come out purple, swollen, squished, angry, and with a head shaped like a cone. When you first see your child, "beautiful" is probably not the adjective that will come to mind. But don't worry—once they are cleaned up, fed, and swaddled, and their cone is covered with a hat, you will have the cutest baby around.

11. You delivered the baby, the end. In the movies the mom goes into labor, the baby comes out, she holds the baby with a rapturous look on her face, and then we fast-forward and suddenly everyone is back at home together, the end. But what about everything that happens in between? What the movies don't tell you is that between those last two events, you're going to have to spend one to three days hanging out in the hospital. I never knew how important those days were until I experienced them—and I have to tell you, even though delivery-room nurses are phenomenal, it's pretty messed up that they get all of the credit, because the postnatal nurses are equally great, and they are crazy helpful in those first few days after giving birth. They should get more screen time, because they are saints. My husband and I are very intelligent people, but taking care of a newborn was not part of our knowledge base. So our initial days as caretakers of a newborn were like parenting boot camp. The postnatal nurses helped us learn to do everything for the first time. Without them, we would have been lost. You will enter a nervous novice and leave a competent (albeit terrified) parent in the following areas:

- How to hold the baby
- When to feed the baby
- How to hold the baby while feeding
- How to burp the baby
- How to change a diaper
- How often to change a diaper
- How to avoid being peed on
- How to put the baby to sleep
- How to swaddle
- How to soothe a crying baby
- How to care for the umbilical cord
- How to take care of a circumcision (if you choose to go this route)
- How to put a baby in a car seat

Believe it or not, the list goes on. Even after the three-day crash course, all I could think was, *Are you really trusting me to take this thing home?*

(The Mommy Gene)

As mentioned before, the whole "mom" thing was never really something I felt predisposed to do—so when I found out I was pregnant for the first time, I felt shock well before the excitement kicked in. In my mind, there were the women with the "mommy gene"—the ones born to take care of children. Think Susie Homemaker, June Cleaver, or Alice from *The Brady Bunch*—women who as little girls played with dolls and dreamt of the day they would become mothers; women who love to hold babies, even other people's; women who are really good at scrap booking. And then there were the other women—women like me.

I have always been a bit of a tomboy, and honestly I wasn't quite sure I even wanted children before I had them. As a result of this, on the day I went in to deliver my first child, I was a nervous wreck. What if this was a huge mistake? What if not having the "mommy gene" would make me a bad mother?

Luckily, everything changed once my child was placed in my arms. As if on cue, some internal switch flipped and I did something completely out of character—I whipped out my tit in front of everyone and set to work getting him to latch on.

Who is this person? I wondered.

The second I had my first child, some sort of instinct kicked in, and I realized that even though I didn't have the stereotypical makeup of a "natural" mom, I did have the ability to be a good mom. You don't have to want to hold your child all the time, or know how to crochet them a blanket—you just have to love and take care of them, in whatever way you know how.

Just as a heads up, some moms who experience postpartum depression may feel uncomfortable, anxious, or even repulsed at the thought of even touching their child after they give birth. If that's the case for you, know that you are not alone; many other mothers and even fathers have gone through this. In most cases these feelings are temporary, however if you notice the baby blues have not gone away after two-to-three weeks, you should consult a doctor.

(My Baby Blues)

As like most things under the pregnancy umbrella, postpartum depression was another thing I was totally unprepared for. It doesn't help that this is not a baby
related topic that comes up in most social circles. Therefore, I thought I would share my experience with you.

I ended up going through postpartum depression following the births of both of my children. Surprisingly, I
didn't actually know I had it with my first child. Instead
of feeling upset or sad, as the name suggests, I only had
symptoms of anxiety—but my anxiety had nothing to do
with my baby. Instead, the main triggers were my husband,
housework, and my job.

My husband chose to be a stay-at-home dad, which was a big adjustment for him. After a few weeks of trading in his autonomy for no sleep, diapers, puke, and a screaming infant, he clearly wasn't as happy-go-lucky of a guy as he was pre-baby, which makes perfect sense. However at the time I felt like I was to blame for this change in mood, so I made it my mission to make sure he was "doing okay" every day. Looking back I probably annoyed the heck out of him, as he most likely just needed some time alone. Go away neurotic mommy, and please take crying baby with you!

And then there was the constant cleaning. When you get to a later chapter in this book, called Housework Multiplier, you will find that maintaining a clean house while raising a baby is impossible. There will always be more laundry and dishes to do. This posed a major problem for me in the months after giving birth, because my anxiety would sky rocket if I walked into a messy house after work. I literally felt it in my bones. The angst wouldn't subside until everything was cleaned up and back in its place.

Finally, my job. As if trying to keep a happy husband, clean home and being a new mommy wasn't enough, going back to work in a competitive sales environment only worsened my anxiety. Even today, I'm still conflicted with feelings about being a "bad mom" for choosing to exceed at my career instead of stay at home. At the height of my postpartum I remember not being able to sleep at night, because I couldn't stop stressing that I wasn't high enough up on my company's sales leader report. I spent the better part of a year staring at the ceiling worrying that I wasn't good enough.

Writing all of this down now sounds absolutely crazy, but as mentioned before I didn't end up putting two and two together until the postpartum went away. One day, about nine months after giving birth, I woke up and felt like an entirely new person. My mind and my body were refreshed. Since I had previously felt nothing but angst for such a long period of time, my new-found composure was noticeable. Even walking downstairs and discovering that all of the previous night's dishes were still in sink didn't get me going. It turns out the postpartum had ended, and my constant anxiety went with it. Good bye baby blues, welcome back normal self

Luckily with my second child I knew what to expect. As soon as the anxiety returned I went to see a doctor. I ended up trying a few types of anti-anxiety medications, but didn't stick with them for long. They actually worked too well; I found myself without a care in the world. That is a great feeling to have if you are all alone relaxing on a tropical island, however it is not so good if you have to juggle being a mom with a high-octane career. Again the anxiety lasted about nine months, but at least this time I knew what was happening and that there was light at the end of the tunnel.

(Breast-Feeding)

Breast-feeding gets its own chapter because it's such a controversial subject. Here's my take on the whole thing: Yes, the American Academy of Pediatrics recommends breast-feeding for at least the first six months. But you need to do what's right for you and your baby. Allergies, work schedules, personal preferences, and a slew of other factors may make bottle-feeding a better option for you—and if that's the case, you shouldn't feel weird or guilty or ashamed about it.

When I found out I was pregnant, I decided I would go with the tatas. (It didn't hurt that I'd heard all about how you could burn thousands of calories by breast-feeding.)

And I just assumed it would be simple enough, so I didn't give it much more thought than that. But boy, was I wrong. Breast-feeding isn't nearly as easy as I was led to believe—but by the time I realized that, I was already in the thick of battle.

I wouldn't want anyone else to go into things as unprepared as I was, so here's a list of everything you should know about breast-feeding before your little one comes screaming into the world, demanding food.

1. **Breast milk versus formula:** In the first few days after delivery, moms produce colostrum—a high-concentrate, yellow liquid rich in antibodies and anti-bacterials that help strengthen your baby's immune system and helps them perform their first bowel movement. Actual breast milk doesn't start coming in until two to three days after delivery. There's some evidence to suggest that babies who are breast-fed are less likely to die of sudden infant death syndrome (SIDS) and have a lower likelihood of developing diabetes, asthma, high cholesterol, and even leukemia. Score for breast-feeding. But bottle-fed babies get the advantage of bonding with both parents, as your partner can help with the feedings, and because formula isn't digested as easily as breast milk, babies who drink formula stay fuller longer. Another bonus for moms who

go the formula route is that they can eat whatever they want, not to mention have a glass of wine without worrying about exposing their child to alcohol. So clearly there are pros and cons to both approaches. You'll figure out pretty quickly what works best for you and your baby, so don't let guilt force a choice that doesn't suit you.

2. **Positioning:** If you are a first-time mom, positioning your baby to breast-feed is actually quite tricky. You just learned how to hold your infant two minutes ago, and now you have to face-plant them into your chest. A word of advice: If you are struggling, throw all modesty out the door and ask for help. Invite a nurse or lactation specialist to come to your aid. They will help get you and your baby into a comfortable feeding position, and they'll educate you about the ins and outs of breast-feeding. I should warn you, however, that lactation nurses can be pretty intense. My lactation nurse, Ulga (not her real name, but she looked like an Ulga—she was a giant of a woman), manhandled the crap out my boobs to get my child to latch on. I don't regret enlisting her, because in the end her advice helped get the job done. But it was quite an experience. And another thing about lactation nurses: many are very pro-breast-feeding and very

anti-formula. Again, don't let them make you feel bad or push you into something you're not comfortable with. If you've thought things through and decided on formula, stick to your guns.

3. **Engorged breasts:** "Engorged" is not a friendly term when it comes to describing your boobs, and believe me, it's not a fun feeling. But it happened to me with both of my children, and it could very well happen to you. Basically, having engorged breasts means that your boobs have gotten so big and swollen that your child can't latch on to your nipple—which, in turn, means they can't eat. And babies eat a ton the first few weeks, so this quickly becomes a problem. This was a huge cause of frustration for me with my first child; I was under the assumption that breast-feeding would be easy. You simply place your nipple into your baby's mouth, and they go to town. But I had a new problem on my hands. As soon as my baby was born, my tits exploded from size E to size Z! My breast tissue completely dwarfed the size of my nipples, so our baby couldn't latch. As a result, I had to pump out the milk and feed my child with a syringe until the swelling went down. With my second child, I found a better solution than the pump-and-syringe-feed method—little cups

called breast shells. You place them over your areolas, and the cups gradually pull your nipple out, providing a larger place for your baby to latch. There's also another nifty tool called a guard—basically a plastic pasty with holes that will keep your child from slipping off your nipple while he or she eats—that works wonders. "Engorged," "breast shells," "nipple guards" . . . seriously? Yeah. I told you breast-feeding wasn't that easy.

4. **Pain:** Breast-feeding is like having someone put clothespins on your nipples eight times a day. Believe me, this is not an exaggeration. And I'm not telling you out of a twisted desire to scare you out of breast-feeding—I just think everyone should know what they're getting into. When it's time to eat, your baby goes from precious newborn to ravenous zombie in 1.5 seconds. They start thrashing around, mouth open wide, until they find what they are looking for—your vulnerable nipple—and then, when the food source has been identified, they clamp down with all their might and will not let go. Ouch! Luckily, the pain should only occur on the initial latch. If it continues to hurt while your baby is feeding, then he or she may have latched on wrong. If this happens, pull the kid off—if you can—and try to start over. The larger

your child opens on the way in, the better, because you want them getting the whole nipple in their mouth, not just the tip. If you've tried and tried and are still having trouble, call a nurse and they'll help you out. I was surprised to find out that lactation specialists even do house calls. The second thing you want to do to limit your pain is take constant care of your valuable nips. After every feed, wipe down your nipples and then lather them with lanolin. This will help soothe them from the attack you just endured, as well as prevent drying, cracking, and bleeding.

5. **With pain comes gain:** There are two major benefits to breast-feeding. One is for your baby: Breast milk can provide your child with the essential nutrients and vitamins they will need to grow and thrive. Studies also show that breast milk can prevent your baby from contacting a series of illnesses at the start of their fragile lives. The other is for you: Breast-feeding is a workout for the body. You can burn up to five hundred calories a day breast-feeding—something that, as I mentioned before, I was very happy to hear. I promise you, when you see what your stomach looks like after giving birth, you will be all for burning the extra calories. The downside is that this constant working out can

cause fatigue. I addressed this by setting up two main feeding stations in my house—one next to the couch and one next to my bed—where I kept bottles of water and small snacks like crackers and trail mix. Try it! It helps keep you going and the breast milk flowing (poet).

6. **It's all fun and games until you squirt your child in the eye:** Breast milk gets everywhere! You will have it all over you, all over your baby, on the bed, on the chair, on the floor, everywhere—and there's nothing you can do about it. Sometimes when those boobs get going, they just don't stop. Remember the scene in *Austin Powers* when the Fembots are spraying bullets from their boobs? That's a pretty accurate depiction of what can happen with your breast milk. On multiple occasions, I have pulled my baby off to burp him, and the milk has come flying out and shot him in the face. And I promise you, they do not like it when you squirt them in the eye with breast milk. I strongly advise you to keep as many blankets, towels, and burp cloths as possible nearby when you are feeding; you'll need them. Also, make sure to wear breast pads in between feedings. If you don't, you'll be walking around with two wet dots on your shirt all day long.

7. **Pumpin':** If you are breast-feeding you are probably pumping. I never knew what it was like to feel like a Dairy cow until the day I hooked myself up to a breast pump. For some reason I was very comfortable using a breast pump from the start, but a lot of women find them intimidating. And for good reason. First of all, the machine looks and sounds like a small torture device. Second, when you look down at those suction cups and see that your nipples are being stretched to three inches long, there are just no words. At least it's less painful than the Jaws of Life your baby comes equipped with.

8. **Coffee milk:** Everything you eat and drink can affect your breast milk. Spicy food, coffee, and alcohol are the ones that seem to be discussed the most. I knew about spicy food and alcohol (I avoided the first and just "pumped and dumped" when I had the second), but coffee caught my husband and me completely by surprise. This is how it went down: I pumped a lot in the beginning of my pregnancy to create a solid milk supply—you know, so my husband could share in the fun of the middle-of-the-night feedings—and one night when we gave the baby a bottle of stored milk, instead of him falling back to sleep like normal, the opposite happened. He was wide-eyed, arms and legs kicking, no signs

of being even remotely close to slumber. *Why is our child acting like he's just had a double shot of espresso?* I wondered—and then it hit me. I had pumped that morning right after drinking one of those crack lattes I'm so fond of and popped the milk in the fridge. That same milk was now running through our child's tiny body. We had just given him a full-on caffeine buzz. Whoops. Moral of the story: label your milk!

9. **It's okay to throw in the towel:** If you find that breast-feeding just isn't for you, or that you're not producing enough milk to keep up with your growing baby, don't worry. It is *perfectly fine* to go the formula route. Also, some babies are just born with a sensitivity to milk. My first child ended up being lactose intolerant, which meant that he was sensitive to both my breast milk and formula. After weeks of him crying twenty hours a day, we gave him away. Just kidding—we were saved by soy milk. To this day, he is on soy and almond milk. So once again, do what is right for you and what is right for your baby!

PART THREE:

(Get Ready for Your Life to Change)

Everyone will tell you that having children will change your life, not to mention your body—and they are 100 percent correct. My husband and I often lie in bed talking about this subject. It is definitely bittersweet. We love our children and would never take back our decision to have them. But we still miss the days when we could do anything we wanted to—the years when no one was depending on us for anything.

Once you have children, the simple freedoms you took for granted in your pre-baby life become very clear—for instance, going to the bathroom alone, leaving your house in a timely manner, and having boobs that don't sag to your belly button.

I wish someone had prepped me in advance so I would have been prepared for some of the more dramatic transitions that would occur when I started the baby-having process. But I guess my friends and family didn't want to scare me out of it.

The next part of this book covers just a few of the post-baby life and bodily changes that I was not quite ready for. Hopefully knowing about them ahead of time will help you adjust more quickly than I did!

(The Constipation Continues)

Many people don't like the sensation of torture, so they take pain medication during and after the birth of their babies. I am one of those people. What I was unaware of beforehand, however, is that pain medication can lead to constipation. And I'm not just talking wait-out-the-day constipation—no, I'm talking a full week of no release.

Following the birth of both of my children, going number two became quite the epic event. I would spend up to an hour just sitting on the toilet, waiting for something to happen—and even after all that, I usually left the bathroom defeated, stomach aching, the red imprints of the toilet seat on my bottom. (Added bonus: All the pushing made my butt button return full force).

One particularly bad case of constipation came following the birth of our second baby. Even though I hadn't gone to the bathroom in days, I woke up excited because we were going to have some of our first non-grandparent company come by for a visit. Unfortunately, by the time our two friends arrived I was already camped out in the bathroom, engaged in an epic battle with a poop that just would not come all the way out. (I guess the appropriate word here is "turtle head"?)

"Hello!" I said from behind the closed bathroom door when they arrived.

Then my husband took them into the living room, and they met our newest addition and visited for a while, and then it was time for them to go—and I was still on the toilet.

"Good-bye!" I said from behind the closed bathroom door as they left.

Mega-sized, stubborn poop: 1. Me and my butt: 0.

Even though constipation is a very normal side effect of having a baby, no one said anything about it to me in advance. A simple, "Hey, PS, your as* is going to shutdown after your baby is born," would have been really nice—but no such luck. As a result, I didn't exactly know what do when it happened, so I went with a trial-and-error method.

Here's what I've discovered about constipation remedies after two pregnancies:

1. **Over-the-counter laxatives (pill form):** I would not recommend these. They took a long time to work and made my stomachache even worse.

2. **Non-oral laxatives:** "Non-oral" is nice way of saying you have to insert them up your own anal cavity. Seems a bit counterintuitive, I know. Why would you put something inside your butt when the whole problem is that there's too much stuff in there in the first place, right? But I'm telling you, they work. You will find the process a bit awkward and really gross. But it's worth it. Non-oral laxatives are fast acting and they don't increase your stomach pain the way the oral ones do.

3. **MiraLAX:** Recommend to me by my mother, Mira-LAX became my saving grace in the few weeks after my baby was born. I was a little concerned about pouring so much of this mysterious white powder into a glass of water and then downing it, but was happy to find out it is completely tasteless and painless. It doesn't act as fast as the non-oral laxatives, but it does make eliminations easier going forward—and you don't have to shove it up your bum.

Important note: If none of the above remedies work, you should probably go see your doctor!

The Arrival of the Stomach Flap

As I mentioned before, the baby bump can be very flattering—especially midway through pregnancy, before your face and ankles swell up. At that point your little basketball is perfectly round and you look cute in everything you wear.

Sadly, that phase doesn't last long. Once your child is born, that basketball pops and a saggy flap of leftover skin takes its place.

I was totally taken off guard by my post-baby stomach. Honestly, I was appalled. During my pregnancy, I'd never really thought about what would happen to my body after the baby was born; I just figured the baby came out and presto, change-o, my belly would go back to normal. But no—instead of returning to its pre-baby shape, my belly had transformed into a flabby, stretched-out mess.

I first noticed this at the hospital but figured I was just swollen and it would eventually flatten out. Sadly, as the swelling went down over the next few weeks, instead of my tummy getting flatter, the stretched out skin bulge just became more pronounced.

To make matters worse, I realized this new shape created quite the clothing dilemma. I was now too small to fit into my maternity clothes (except for the rubber band jeans, which I wore for like a full year after having my first baby and am currently still wearing 6 months after having baby number two), but too large for my pre-baby wardrobe. I was also exhausted all of the time from being up all night, so the last thing I wanted to do was get out there and get my body back into shape. Would this extra patch of skin ever go away?

The best advice and reassurance someone gave me was to apply the forty-week rule to your body: You had forty weeks to put the weight on, so give yourself forty weeks (or more like a year, in my case) to take it off. Try not to stress, because unless you are crazy genetically gifted (or loaded and can afford the training or surgery), your stomach is not going to flatten overnight. Give yourself some time and ease back into working out. You may never wear a bikini again, but eventually your stomach will look better than it does now.

(The Case of the
Disappearing Boobs)

I was finally getting used to having torpedoes by the time my first child was born, and I hoped my new large and perky ta tas were there to stay.

No such luck. Once the milk dried up, my boobs did as well. Just like with my stomach, all that remains now are two saggy sacks of excess skin, covered in stretch marks. Hot, right?

Even if someone had told me I would be pulling my boobs out of my armpits for the rest of my life, I still would have gone through with the decision to breast-feed my kids. The bonding it allowed me to have with them when they were tiny infants is a memory I still look back on fondly. But sadly, the insecure part of me has trouble looking in the mirror at what is left of my chest to this day. I am still seriously contemplating some sort of lift or implants. (Please, no judging.)

In the meantime, I am glad that the bra has come a long way since its early days. A good bra can be an effective solution for your post-baby boobs. Once I realized I wasn't getting my E's back, I went out and spent a good amount of money on some quality support. And what do you know, with the help of some underwire, my boobs actually can pass as somewhat perky again. Nobody (except for my husband, and now everyone who has read this book) would even be able to tell the difference.

(Sayonara, Sleep)

Sleep? What is that? Here I go again, talking about it. I think some part of me is convinced that if I keep talking about it, I may actually get some.

It's hard for me to remember the last time I actually had a full nights' sleep, because I am currently back in the twilight zone, waking up at all hours of the night to have my nipples pinned and poop shot at me. Not fun.

Unfortunately, there is not a lot you can do to prepare yourself for what no sleep feels like. The best advice I can give you is that if you are pumping, and your baby is willing to take a bottle, you should have your partner step up to the plate on occasion. In our case, my husband would take all of the feeds until midnight, and then I would take over from there until morning. It helped a little.

Another thing you can do to get some extra Z's is try to nap when your baby naps. Full disclosure: I failed at this. I always felt like I had too much to do between catching up on work and the household chores, so I usually opted for writing e-mails and cleaning over shut-eye. This of course made me even more exhausted than I was before. As if on cue, when I was finally done with my work and ready for a quick nap, my baby would wake up.

Even though the napping-while-baby-naps thing didn't work for me, you should totally give it a go—who knows, it might work for you!

Eventually the initial shock of insomnia will wear off, and you will fall into a walking dead–like routine. Then, when you think you can't possibly go another night without rest, your child will decide to sleep through the night. I know this sounds magical, but it's a mixed blessing: it's what you have been waiting for, but the first time (possibly the first couple of times) it happens, it will scare the heck out of you. You will panic, thinking there is something wrong with your child, and you will go dashing into their room to make sure they're still breathing.

I remember the first time our oldest child almost slept through the night. I woke up around four in the morning and discovered that the monitor, which hadn't been plugged in, had run out of batteries. *Holy crap, did the baby wake up and I missed it? Is he okay?* I was freaking out.

I quickly got up, went into the baby's room, and peered into the crib. He was there, sleeping safe and sound—but I must not have been as quiet as I thought, because his little eyes popped open the second I bent over him. I instinctively hit the deck and proceeded to army crawl out of his nursery, hoping I had not been spotted. No such luck. He started crying, and soon the whole house was awake. If I had just let him be, he would have successfully slept through the night for the very first time!

Eventually your house will establish a healthier sleeping routine and your body and your brain will start to feel normal. That is, until you decide to have another child, and then you will have to go through the torture session all over again.

(The Decline of Your Social Life)

Once you have a child, your adult life as you knew it will be changed forever. Since we were in our mid-twenties when we had our first child, my husband and I both took this one pretty hard. No more after-work cocktail hours. No more romantic late-night dinner dates. No more Ninja Turtle beer pong tournaments. We had no idea how selfish we were until someone even more selfish entered the world and started demanding all our time. I think this ended up being a plus for my liver, but a total negative for our social skills. We definitely turned into a pair of hermits for the first few months after our child was born.

Eventually, we got enough guts to venture out into society, but in a much tamer fashion than we had before. To this day, if we take the kids out to dinner with us, we go early. It is usually just us and the blue-hairs—which is perfect, because they tend to love children. I think they are so old they have forgotten how hard it is to actually raise little ones.

When we are at dinner, the goal is to cause as little of a scene as possible. (You're welcome, pre-baby, romantic couples who want to eat in peace at 7:30 P.M.) This usually means we sit down, quickly scan the menu, and order everything the second the server appears. Once the food is brought to the table, we request to pay the check—that way if either of our ticking time bombs go off while we are actually eating, we can head for the door. I also recommend dining at restaurants that have outside seating; this allows the volume of your table to be less noticeable.

We're the first of our circle of friends to have little ones—which basically means that when we're getting ready to go to bed, our friends are just getting ready to go out.

After having our first kid, almost every weekend we would get an invitation to some sort of social gathering. Meet you for dinner at 8:00 P.M.? Sorry, no can do—that's the baby's bedtime. Girl's night out at 9:00 P.M.? Wish I could, but I'm totally exhausted—rain check? Clubbing at 10:00 P.M.? Zzzzzzzz . . .

After a few months of declining all invitations taking place after dusk, we just stopped getting invited out altogether. Some people may feel bummed out by being excluded from their former social scene, but I honestly felt relief. I was so tired all the time; all I wanted to do at the end of the day was pass out on the couch.

Somewhere around the fourth month PB (post baby) our lives as antisocial husband and wife started to get a little old. There is only so much you, your spouse, and a non-verbal infant can talk about. We had to seek out adult interaction. And since our friends without children weren't willing to meet us out earlier, we realized we would have to find new acquaintances in a similar situation to our own.

This seclusion then re-emergence into society will most likely happen to you as well. If you are like us and don't have anyone in your current social circle with young ones, seeking out new friends to share your plight with is actually not that hard to do.

Start by going to places where parents with little children will be. Day care, the park, the children's museum, assorted playgroups, insane asylums . . . you get the point. The great part about meeting people with kids the same age as yours is you will be instantly bonded by your parallel tales of woe.

These are people who won't get offended when you have to leave because it's naptime or because one of your kids just bit someone. You can go ahead and change a diaper in front of them without them looking at you in disgust. And they'll want to do dinners early too, which is great, because it means you can socialize and still get home in time for baths, bed, and *Jeopardy.*

(The Decline of Your Sex Life)

Many people joke that marriage ends your sex life, but that's a lie—in our case, anyway. Marriage didn't end our sex life. Babies did.

Here's the thing: After spending your whole day listening to your child crying, changing diapers, and having your boobs accosted every other hour, sex is the last thing you want. By the time evening comes, you're exhausted, and you probably haven't even had time to take a shower, let alone get in the mood. It's easy to see why your romantic life takes a backseat.

I wrote in the beginning of this book that I wasn't going to tell you "had" to do anything, but I am going to take that part back for this chapter, because there is one thing you have to do: you have to get the sexual part of your relationship up and running again after your baby is born.

Yes, immediately following giving birth, you may not be up for sex. It makes sense: your hormones have been hijacking your body for the better part of a year, and your lady bits have just been roughed up pretty badly. But you can't forget about your relationship with your partner. Keeping the spark alive is very, very important.

Here are a few things that can help get you back in the mood again after having a baby.

1. **Go on dates ALONE.** It is amazing how relaxing and slow-paced the meal can be without a disaster waiting to happen sitting in a baby carrier next to you.

2. **Don't wait until the end of the day to have sex.** This is usually when you are the most tired. After playing mom all day, it is very easy to choose the couch and a movie over the bed and a bang. So go for it earlier in the day—right after you wake up in the morning or during your kid's afternoon nap are two good options!

3. **Try and shake up the venue.** The bedroom is cozy, but why not try out the shower or the dining room table?

4. **Read a romance novel.** I, like many of you, recently read a popular novel with the word "grey" in the title, and it worked like a charm. My husband didn't even know what hit him. (It was a black leather paddle—just kidding. Maybe.)

5. **Take one for the team.** Even if you're not in the mood for sex, sometimes it's good to just do it anyway. You will be surprised how quickly your attitude can change once things get going.

For my husband and I, having sex again was incredibly important, because for a while PB, everything was about the "B" and no longer about us. We were two separate people trying to make it through the longest parenting days ever, just so we could fall asleep and start all over again. I could see a routine forming that was pushing us apart and I didn't like it.

So, one day, even though no part of my body wanted to be intimate, I brought my husband up into our bedroom and we had sex. The experience was much more for his benefit than mine, but sex triggers endorphins, so I left the room feeling genuinely improved as well. From that point on, we both got better about taking time to be together. After all, in eighteen years (hopefully) our children will be out of the house and it will just be the two of us left. We need to keep the romance alive so we can continue to enjoy our lives together when the nest is empty.

(The Decline of Hangovers)

I don't even remember the last time I had a hangover—and that's something I never thought I'd say. But guess what? I don't miss them one bit.

It's not that I suddenly stopped liking the taste of alcohol as soon as I had a baby. It's that I learned pretty fast that having a hangover with a baby is way, way worse than having a hangover without one. Unlike in your pre-baby days, when you could just wallow in your own misery for an entire afternoon bingeing on leftover Chinese food, hangovers are no longer allowed once you are a parent. Your child does not care if you have a headache or if you want to vomit every time you stand up. They still expect to be fed, changed, held, played with, and soothed.

This probably seems like common sense, but I warn you to steer clear of the excess partying anyway. If you are like me, there will be a moment after you have a baby that you get caught up in the excitement of being out and about without your child. It is amazing how carefree you can feel when you don't have to worry about the next diaper change. And the more relaxed you start to feel, the higher the potential for hangover slip-up.

This happened to me about six months after having my first child. My in laws came into town and offered to watch our child overnight so my husband and I could get a much-needed break. Instead of choosing a romantic dinner with just the two of us, we decided to go out with some of our rugby friends.

If you have not been around rugby players before, they are some of the nicest people you'll ever meet, but they are also some of the wildest. They love playing rugby, playing rugby while drinking beer, singing songs, singing songs while drinking beer, and dressing up in odd themed costumes—you guessed it—while drinking beer.

This particular night was pirate themed. So there we were at the bar with some of our best friends, dressed up like a couple of buccaneers, and after a while I started to get caught up in the excitement of being out of the house for once without our little one. It was just so nice to finally have some adult freedom. So nice that, in my infinite wisdom, I thought it would be a great idea to toast to the occasion. Shots for everyone!

One shot turned into two, of course, and two turned into too many. The next thing I fully remember is waking up in our hotel room, still dressed as a pirate, with the worst hangover in the history of hangovers. My head was pounding, I was sweating profusely, and the room smelled like vomit. The smell made sense when I realized there was puke all over my pirate costume.

When I asked my husband what happened, he told me that after one of the many shots I had taken, I turned my head to the side and casually puked all over myself. That's when he escorted me out of the bar and back to our hotel.

Once I had cleaned myself up that morning, we went home and I was forced right back into the routine of caring for a little one. I felt like I was going to die, but parenting came first. It was terrible.

My body didn't fully recover until a few days later. My tolerance for drinking had gotten pretty low, but my recovery abilities, it seemed, were even worse. Lesson learned. Argggh, matey!

Today when my friends want to get together for cocktails, I keep the intake to a minimum and I absolutely steer clear of all shots. Also, if it's a weekend, I find having a few drinks during the day to be much easier. That way I am in bed at a decent hour and ready to parent the second the 2:00 A.M., 4:00 A.M., and 6:00 A.M. baby alarms go off.

(From Politics to Poop)

You know how you and your partner like to
have conversations about adult things, like current events
and politics? Well, prepare to say good-bye to those conversations once you have a baby, and hello to poop.

The reason for this is simple: babies poop a lot. Which
means you're dealing with it on a day-to-day (hour-to-
hour) basis once your child arrives in the world. And when
this happens, weirdly, all of a sudden the color, smell, and
texture of poop all become quite interesting.

Personally, I got obsessed with my baby's poop the second I saw meconium in his diaper. Meconium, if you don't

know this already (and why would you?), is this black stuff that babies poop out not long after birth. And man was I shocked when I saw that gem in my baby's diaper. Why was it so dark?

The next poop to expect after the meconium is the liquid gold kind. Luckily it doesn't have much of a smell, but it does seem to always—always—be in your baby's diaper, and up their back, when you open it. It's a quick trip from mouth to rear with a newborn. And warning: Boy babies may be more likely to pee on you, but all babies have the ability to shoot poop at you.

I was reminded of this recently in the middle of the night as I was changing my newborn. He clenched his little buns together and shot his poop right at me. If there was a contest for doo-doo distance, he would have placed on this one. I was covered! There was so much poop on me, I had to wake up my husband (though he was probably awake already, because I screamed when the poop hit me) to finish changing the baby's diaper so I could clean myself up.

After liquid gold come the stinky sh*ts. If you are using formula, or when you start basic foods, the poop changes yet again, to brown and smelly. The real stuff. This is when my husband and I started playing, rock-paper-scissors to see whose turn it would be to change the diaper. This is also when you will start minding which trash can you put your baby's soiled diaper in.

Imagine if baby books actually told you the truth about baby poop. Congratulations on your newborn, you will now be looking at, smelling, and touching your child's feces multiple times a day for the next four to five years. That's 1,825 days of being up close and personal with poop. Fun!

(Code Red)

Eventually, you will find that changing five to ten diapers a day will become instinctual, and you'll fall into a comfortable baby-changing routine—until, that is, you experience your first "Code Red." At which point everything falls apart.

I always check on my kids before going to bed. It lets me rest easier knowing they are tucked in and sound asleep. And usually it's just a quick peek in and I'm done. But one night, as I was performing my regular bed check rounds, I realized something just wasn't right. Before I even opened our two-year-old's door, I could smell it: he had pooped in his sleep.

This, of course, presented a dilemma. I didn't want to leave him lying in his own filth, but I really didn't want to risk waking him up either. Every part of me wanted to turn around, ignore the stench, and go to bed. But letting a child slumber in a pile of poop is probably not the best parenting decision, not to mention the fact that it would lead to massive diaper rash that I would also have to deal with. So I had no other choice: I had to order the "Code Red."

Below are the step-by-step procedures for properly handling a Code Red:

1. Enter room quietly and keep lights as low as possible.

2. Lay out towel and diapers, and pull out the correct amount of wipes in advance to keep noise to a minimum. It is best to overestimate the amount of wipes needed.

3. Lift child from bed as gently as possible and lay them down on the towel.

4. Remove soiled diaper. (Caution: Try not to gag out loud.)

5. Gently clean soiled area. Slightly more elbow grease may be required if the poop has been in the

diaper for a while, but refrain from applying too much pressure.

6. If your child stirs, try and shush them back to sleep.

7. Place clean diaper on child.

8. Replace child's PJ bottoms. If you think this will result in waking them up, abort PJ bottom replacement—it's not worth it.

9. Channel your inner David Copperfield and levitate your child back to their bed.

10. Close door. If Code Red has been successfully completed, fist pump, then wash hands and go to bed.

*(**Note:** A Code Red is best done as a two-man job. If you are forced to go it alone . . . Godspeed and good luck.)*

(Sick Baby)

No matter how hard you try, you cannot prevent babies and children from getting sick. I knew there would be a day when illness would hit our household, but that doesn't mean my husband and I were actually prepared for it—and even if we had been, it still would have sucked.

Our first major round was with a little something called the croup, which I honestly thought was an ailment that children only got back in the days of *Little House on the Prairie.*

Instead of "croup," I like to call it the "oh my god, my baby is suffocating sickness." It happened when our firstborn was around five months old. We woke up to what sounded like the barking of a seal mixed with a baby's cry over the monitor, and I rushed to the crib to find our son barely able to breath and hot to the touch. I picked him up to soothe him, but every time I thought he was about to stop crying, he would choke, scare himself, and start to wail again.

Being a first-time mom, I had no clue what to do when this happened, so I resorted to FTMEP (First-Time Mom Emergency Protocol):

Step 1: Page the pediatrician and nervously wait for call back.

Step 2: Call Mom, wake her up from a sound sleep, and ask for advice.

Step 3: Look up all symptoms on the Internet and scare yourself and your mom even more.

Step 4: Tell Mom you have to call her back because the doctor is calling in.

Step 5: Be talked off the ledge by the pediatrician as he or she recites the diagnosis.

Step 6: Send husband out immediately to get prescription.

Step 7: Forget to call Mom back. (Have no fear; she will call you back again and again until you pick up and tell her what is actually wrong with her grandchild.)

Even with the medication in our son's system, the rest of the evening was terrible. We put him into a bath to cool his temp then held him outside of a hot shower to breathe the steam—and all the while, the baby seal kept crying. By the time he finally fell asleep on my chest, the sun was coming up.

Croup: 1. Parents: 0.

A few days later, I told another parent the harrowing tale of that night's events, and she looked at me as if those traumatic eight hours were just a walk in the park.

"Yeah, we went through that too," she said. "It's pretty normal for babies to get."

Did everyone know about croup but us?

Unfortunately croup was not the only sickness to rear its ugly head in our household. My husband and I had to go through quite a few more moments of panic before we got accustomed to the fact that no matter how hard we tried to keep them healthy, our kids were going to get sick.

I have shared a few of the more common illnesses below. You will still get scared out of your mind the first time your child gets one of these, and you will still need to consult a doctor for proper diagnosis, but at least you will know you are not alone.

- **Roseola.** Sudden, high fever—we're talking 102, 103—accompanied by a body rash. Our first born got this when he was eighteen months old and I was pregnant with our second child. I was already a hormonal mess, so when I saw the results on the thermometer, I skipped FTMEP and immediately packed up and headed to the hospital. It turned out I'd overreacted slightly. The doctor on duty simply prescribed Tylenol and a cold bath and sent us home.

- **Respiratory Syncytial Virus (RSV).** Common cold or flu-like symptoms leading to respiratory issues such as wheezing. Our second child came down with this one. By that point we were pretty good at spotting the common cold, but after a week of no improvement in his symptoms, as well as increased difficulty in breathing, we got a little concerned. Our pediatrician diagnosed our son with RSV. Thank god for acronyms, they sound less scary. We ended up having to spend almost an hour holding a nebulizer up to our six month old's mouth at the doctor's office before we were able to pack up and head home.

- **Influenza.** Commonly known as the flu, influenza can cause every crummy symptom imaginable:

fever, runny nose, sore throat, muscle pain, headache, etc. It is pretty much the coup de grâce of
common ailments amongst youngsters. H1N1 happened to be the strain of flu going on at the time,
and although they were vaccinated, both of my
children contracted the flu at the same time. To top
it off, this all went down while my husband and I
were away on vacation. I owe my parents big time;
not only did they spend days nursing our children
back to health, including an overnight at the hospital, they both ended up coming down with the flu
as well. Did I mention grandparents are the best?

Here are a few other common childhood illnesses
that our kids have yet to contract (though I put that up
to luck of the draw, not parenting skill): ringworm, ear
infection, hand, foot, and mouth disease, pink eye, and
the dreaded lice.

You would think hospitals would give new parents a
manual covering the common ailments your child will face
in their first year as a parting gift after delivery—not just
for our peace of mind, but their doctors'. It can't be fun for
them to get frantic calls from new parents all the time. But
until they work that into their routine practices, we'll just
keep FTMEP-ing and hoping for the best.

(Now that I Have a Baby I Wish They Would Invent . . .)

1. **Universal bottles and sippy cups:** There is nothing worse than waking up in the middle of the night to feed your child and trying to find the matching parts to a bottle or a cup. And I always seem to choose wrong. As a result, instead of the milk going into my baby's mouth it leaks out of the sides and all over his face, making for a mess and a screaming baby. Because late-night feedings are so fun even when you don't spill milk everywhere.

2. **Self-snapping baby pajamas:** Whoever thought it was a good idea to create an article of clothing

with fourteen pieces that must be lined up perfectly in order to snap it together *for babies* was a crazy person—or maybe a sadist. You may think I'm exaggerating, but when you're faced with changing a crying, wiggling baby in the middle of the night, putting these pajamas on correctly is basically impossible. No matter how hard you try you will always be left with an extra snap. Don't even bother trying to figure out where you went wrong; it's a losing battle.

3. **Toy remote controls and cell phones that look like the real thing:** Yes, they currently have toy phones and TV remote controls for babies—and they are colorful, light up, and make thousands of interesting sounds. But your baby will not be fooled. The second you are not looking, they will drop the toy remote (or phone) you just handed them and go straight for the real thing. They will then proceed to shove the actual remote (or phone) directly into their mouth to commence a taste test. They know a cheap knock-off when they see one.

4. **An exercise routine for parents and babies:** There never seems to be time to do *anything* once you have a baby, let alone exercise. It would be awesome to have an exercise routine that incorpo-

rates the day-to-day tasks you already do as a parent. For example:

- Strap baby to chest with baby carrier; do twenty squats, rest, and repeat.
- Place baby into swing and push swing back and forth ten times with each arm. Then lie on back and push swing ten times with each leg.
- Breast- or bottle-feed child with one arm and do bicep curls with baby shampoo bottle with the other. Switch after fifteen reps.
- Place baby into seat and play peekaboo while doing sit-ups.
- Place baby into carriage right before naptime and push stroller up and down hills until they fall asleep.

5. **Baby sections on airplanes:** All of our relatives live out of state, which means we have to fly with the kids every time we want to go see them. And when you walk onto the plane with a baby in your arms, you might as well be carrying the plague. Fellow passengers will stare at you in horror, crossing their fingers that you won't sit down anywhere near them. Wouldn't it be amazing to walk into a specially dedicated, fully sanitized section of the

plane filled with other parents who share your plight of flying with an infant? This child-friendly section would come with toys fashioned into the tray tables, children's shows on multiple channels (not just *SpongeBob SquarePants* playing on repeat), an area for walking around, and a bathroom equipped with a changing table larger than a cafeteria tray. Since the airlines have yet to implement these changes, if you find yourself traveling with a baby the below may be of help:

- Avoid late-night flights. I know you think your child will sleep, but they'll probably just cry the entire time (until about two minutes before the plane lands; then he or she will fall fast asleep and you'll bend over backwards trying to get them and your stuff off the plane without waking them.)

- Give your child a bottle during takeoff and landing. This helps with the pressure on their tiny ears.

- Wipe down everything in sight. Kids feel the need to taste every part of the airplane, and who knows what kind of germs are lurking.

- Bring lots of toys, books, and things to do. The used magazine, overhead light switches, tray table, and puke bag are not enough to entertain your child for the entire flight.

- If your child refuses to stop crying, which can happen to even the most seasoned baby flyer, offer to buy the passengers next to you some headphones. That usually takes the glare right off of their faces.

(Post-Baby Phenomena)

1. The "Great Baby Magnet"

After your baby is born, there will be a point when an amazing family member will offer to watch your child for the first time. You will rejoice at the mere prospect of this, and you will look forward to it as the highlight of your week. Then, when the day arrives and you are getting closer to departure time, you will panic.

When my mother offered to watch our son for the first time, I jumped at the chance for a free night out. Between the two of us she was clearly the more practiced parent, but I still felt the need to go over fifty different baby instructions with her before leaving. Then, when it was time to physically walk out the door, I was overcome with the feeling that leaving made me the worst parent in the world.

That feeling didn't dissipate once we were in the car, or even once we got to the restaurant. So, instead of enjoying the evening, I spent the meal texting back and forth with my mom, getting minute-by-minute updates on the baby. I made it through the main course, but we skipped dessert. I had waited all week long to take a mental break, and now I couldn't get home fast enough. Was returning to crying and diaper changing really more appealing than candle-light and crème brûlée?

I can only attribute this to a phenomenon I call the "Great Baby Magnet." You can be having the worst parenting day of your life, but the second you leave your child, you instantly miss them and want to return home to see them. The magnet's effects do eventually lessen— by a few months in I was able to actually enjoy the entire dinner out without the baby—but they are definitely permanent. I can only be gone so long before I am pulled back home.

2. The Housework Multiplier

Before children, I don't remember doing the dishes or washing and folding clothes. I know I must have done these chores, but they were certainly not a major part of my day. Then came Baby #1, and everything changed.

It's seriously like a switch flips: You have a kid, and all of a sudden you are constantly washing bottles and doing laundry. And the older your child gets and the more children you have, the more the housework multiplies. These days, I can clean my house top to bottom and then hours later open my eyes to a sink full of dishes, a mounting load of laundry, and crap everywhere.

If you are a stay-at-home parent and you can afford to get help, you may want to look into getting a housekeeper, at least while the kids are little. Being a parent to young children is the hardest job in the world. There is barely enough time to get dressed and eat, never mind keep the house in order. Don't get upset if you can't get it all done in one day. You are doing your best.

Here are a few things you can look forward to dealing with in your day-to-day cleanup once you have a baby:

- You will wash ten pairs of tiny socks and only find seven in the dryer. The others will have disappeared from the face of the earth.

- When you go to unload the dishwasher, you will find that parts of the baby bottle have slipped through the rack and landed at the bottom during the wash and have now melted into new shapes, never to fit inside of the bottle again.

- You will fill your child's tray with food and rejoice as they eat it all. This illusion will be lost later, as you lift them out of their seat and find all of the food hidden in the high chair and stuck to their butt.

- No matter how hard you try, you will never be able to remove all of the crumbs from the car seat, high chair, and baby stroller.

- You will clean up all of the toys around the house, then a mystery tornado will come through and deposit them right back where they started.

3. The Time Warp

When you have children, time gets warped. All of a sudden the days become very, very long. You wake up at six in the morning to start your routine—and after five diaper changes, three bottles, two naps, and one time out, you look at the clock and it is only two in the afternoon. How can that be? It will feel as if you've been working hard all day, yet in reality only a few hours will have gone by.

By the time our children are in bed, my husband and I are so tired we can barely stay awake to watch TV. A night that I can make it through one thirty-minute sitcom episode is a rarity.

But that's where it gets confusing, because as long as the days are, the opposite is true for the years. You know how everyone—especially the blue-hairs—is always talking about how fast the years go by with kids? They are absolutely correct. I feel like only yesterday, our toddler was just learning to sit up and our newborn was just a blip on the ultrasound screen. I can only imagine how parents feel when they are sending their child off to college.

The best advice I can give is to try and enjoy all of the stages of parenting. (I need to remind myself of this constantly—like when I am on the verge of mental breakdown from my two-year-old throwing an hour-long tantrum). Embrace the good, the bad, and the just plain gross, and don't be in too much of a hurry for your child to grow up—because before you know it, they will.

(Conclusion)

I wish you were a fly on the wall when I was
writing this book, because it would drive home a lot of the
points that I have made. I wrote 30 percent of it standing
up with my youngest strapped to my chest in a baby carrier. I wrote the other 70 percent while constantly being
interrupted to change a diaper, feed a child, send someone
to time out, or keep the entire house from burning down.

Prior to having babies of my own, I had no clue what
pregnancy and parenting were going to be like; therefore it
ended up being trial and error most of the time. My hope
is that this book has prepared you for some of the things
the academic world and your grandmother conveniently

left out. I also hope you were able to get a laugh or two in, especially if you are reading this nine-months pregnant and miserable.

Having kids is awesome, but it is also crazy, stressful, and just plain gross at times. The best thing to do during the tough times is to take a step back and just breathe. (If you're like me you will be also holding a very large glass of red wine while you are doing this.) All parents go through the same things, and you are doing a great job. So enjoy it. After all, the days are long, but the years go by very fast.

Good luck—you'll need it!

(Epilogue)

Fast-forward six months. I am currently sitting on an airplane heading to New Orleans for work, and it feels like this is the only free time I have had to get my final thoughts down on paper. Our youngest son is now seven months old. He has started crawling and his two bottom teeth have come in. Teething babies equal extra tears and less sleep. Luckily, aside from the teeth, he is an incredibly happy baby.

And then there is our first born. He is two and a half, smart as a whip, has the energy of a rabbit, and is full on into the terrible twos. I feel like we are either amazed at or enraged by him, depending on the hour. It is a good thing he is so darned cute. (Yes, even after they're no longer babies, you will feel like your kids are the best-looking ones around.)

Even though I feel like I am constantly stressed out, I could not imagine our lives without our two boys. Or maybe I just tell myself not to remember what pre-baby freedom feels like and to just keep focused on the blessings to come.

Just like with pregnancy, there are so many things that come with parenting that you are totally unprepared for: How long should time-out be? What do you do when someone else's kid hits yours? How do you get a pencil eraser out of a nostril? There are also plenty more laugh-out-loud moments that you are dying to share with others but worry will expose you as a bad parent.

If in the next eighteen years I get an ounce of free time, I will try to record some of the funny little parenting things that my husband and I go through as we raise our kids. At this point, though, I am not too optimistic that I'll ever get free time again—not until our children permanently vacate our home, anyway—so in the event that the next book never makes it down on paper, I will share one final thought:

Being a parent is the toughest job in the world! Children will take all of the energy and patience that you have and then some. Luckily, parenting is also, without a doubt, one of the most rewarding jobs. Even though your kids will not verbalize their thanks, parenting can be rewarded in far better ways. Those rewards come in the form of a smile on their face every time they see you in the morning; watching them complete all of the firsts—first roll over, first sit up, first steps, first driver's license (aah!)— and knowing that the effort you put into raising them will shape them into the people they grow up to be. They are your masterpieces.

May you be blessed with a happy, healthy baby and a loving, participatory partner.

A sense of humor helps too.

(About the Author)

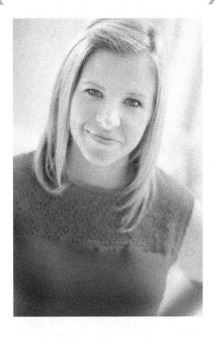

Multitasker extraordinaire **Emily Doherty** is an up-and-coming author, mother of two, and full-time working mom. She is currently a director of mutual fund sales for MFS Investment Management, where she has spent the last eight years educating financial advisors and doing public presentations on the stock market and other investment-related topics. When she is not traveling around the state of Virginia and Washington DC, she is at home with her husband, Patrick, raising their two young sons, Cullen and Lachlan. She equates parenting young boys with controlled chaos and uses their antics for the main inspiration in her books. A graduate of Northeastern University and once an avid rugby player, Doherty is driven to succeed. She looks forward to her upcoming book tours and speaking engagements, and plans to write a series of children's books in the future.

Contact the author at:

Author Emily Doherty

@authoredoherty

Website: www.emilydoherty.com

(About SparkPress)

SparkPress is an independent, hybrid imprint focused on merging the best of the traditional publishing model with new and innovative strategies. We deliver high-quality, entertaining, and engaging content that enhances readers' lives. We are proud to bring to market a list of New York Times bestselling, award-winning, and debut authors who represent a wide array of genres, as well as our established, industry-wide reputation for innovative, creative, results-driven success in working with authors. SparkPress, a BookSparks imprint, is a division o f SparkPoint Studio, LLC.

Learn more at GoSparkPress.com

CPSIA information can be obtained
at www.ICGtesting.com
Printed in the USA
BVHW041155240419
546415BV00008B/361/P